Praise For Reclaimed!

"Through sharing her own personal story, client experiences, and teachings, this book is like walking the path of personal healing hand-in-hand with your best friend. Working with Julie emulates the feeling of a warm comforting hug during a tough time, right before you decide to take the first step towards a positive change."

DR. DENISE PATTERSON, ND

"Julie eloquently guides you home to yourself with her raw vulnerability and an innate ability to help you reclaim the flow of serotonin in the very cells of your soul. You may trust this experienced warrior woman to walk with you as you dive deeply and safely into your personal healing journey. You will never feel alone with Julie by your side."

RUTH VAN DER VOORT, Owner & Director, Yoga Conference & Show

"The world needs more books like *Reclaimed!* Julie is raw, honest, and very inspiring. What I love most is her vulnerable storytelling about life's toughest moments, interwoven with sound practices for reclaiming our lives, healing, and transforming. Julie is a profound teacher and trustworthy guide in the yoga of life and everyday living."

ADRIENNE ENNS, Curator of Joy & CEO at May You Know Joy Inc.

"Julie's journey will empower you to reclaim your story and inspire you to ignite your personal healing process as you root deeply into self-love and self-compassion, gathering the tools you need to weave yourself into wholeness."

NATY HOWARD, Spirit Medicine Healer, Yoga Teacher, Pachakuti Mesa Tradition Mystery School Sanctioned Teacher, and Author of Your Mighty Inner Healer

"Julie's book, *Reclaimed!* is an intimate, raw, real, and compelling account of her own lived experience. It includes rich practical strategies for the woman who wants to live a life of health in all domains of her life; physically, emotionally, intellectual, energetically, and spiritually. Julie's heart is voluminous! She is generous, kind, and overflowing with wisdom. I would highly recommend every woman read this book!"

STEPHANIE ROURKE JACKSON, CEO of Beacon Coaching & Leadership, Speaker, Author

"Julie has created a must-read on how to heal, transform, and reclaim one's life from the inside out. Her book affirms the importance of nurturing and maintaining whole health to encompass the entire Self. This is the key to living a balanced, joyful, and fulfilled life! Julie's love and passion for the care and betterment of her clients is evident. Julie reveals her raw, authentic self to compassionately serve and hold space for others, to let them know they are not alone in their struggles and personal growth journey. *Reclaimed!* is a masterpiece that is sure to inspire and motivate its readers to take care of their whole health with deep passion and love."

GILLIAN SMALL, Transformational Life Coach, Quantum EFT Practitioner, Intuitive Reiki Master, Yoga Instructor, Author

"Julie literally wraps you with love in this book. *Reclaimed!* will open your heart and mind and invite you to connect deeply with your whole being. The combination of her knowledge and willingness to share her story, so transparently, will serve to inspire you in your personal journey of healing and recovery. In such a beautiful way, she speaks to what yoga truly means and the profound impact it can have upon your life, all whilst sharing how it transformed hers. I am so grateful to have Julie in my life, as she empowers and guides me with such passion, love, mindfulness, and kindness. I can assure you she will do the very same for you in the pages of this book!"

TDACHI DENI WHITING, Personal Trainer, Mindset Coach, and Author

"No matter where we may be on our healing journey, physically and mentally-emotionally, Julie has created a safe space for us to land within these pages. As I read *Reclaimed!* what stood out to me most were the testimonials from Julie's clients at the end of every chapter. I found myself rooting for these women, as they shared their successes in working with Julie. In fact, I read *Reclaimed!* in one sitting because I couldn't wait to get to the end of each chapter to celebrate their progress! In sharing her own vulnerability, along with an abundance of tools to support healing, Julie nurtures a strong sense of community throughout this book and reinforces the notion that it truly takes a village to navigate this complex, fragile experience we call life. I felt a spark of empowerment stirring in me from chapter to chapter, and when I finished the book an overwhelming sense of calm settled in. I smiled to myself. For one, I was so damn proud of my friend for doing the dang thing and writing this book! And two, the stories shared in *Reclaimed!* filled me with deep hope and long yearned for inspiration."

ANDREA WETZEL, Team Lead at lululemon

"Julie is a beacon of hope and light that is a true blessing to anyone who engages with her. This book is exactly that. We as women can take on the essence of feeling *less than*. Julie's way of thinking gives us permission to feel and have the confidence in knowing that we are more than enough, despite our past challenges. The power always comes when we decide to reclaim who we have been called to be, no matter what."

BRANDY C. MABRA, CEO, Savvy Clover Coaching & Consulting, Business Coach & Leadership Expert, MHA, ELI-MP, CPC

RECLAIMED!

RECLAIMED!

By Julie Thayer
Foreword by Karen Heaven Claffey
First Edition 2022
Copyright © 2022 Julie Thayer Yoga

Disclaimer
All the information, techniques, skills, and concepts contained within this publication are of the nature of general comment only and are not in any way recommended as individual advice. The intent is to offer a variety of information to provide a wider range of choices now and in the future, recognizing that we all have widely diverse circumstances and viewpoints. Should any reader choose to make use of the information contained herein, this is their decision and the author and publishers do not assume any responsibilities whatsoever under any condition or circumstances.
ISBN: 978-1-7780654-0-8

For more information about the author, Julie Thayer, or for additional trainings, speaking engagements, or media enquiries, please visit: www.juliethayeryoga.com.

Cover design by Ash
Interior design by Ash

Reclaimed!

**A TRANSFORMATIVE YOGA
AND SELF-CARE GUIDE
FOR WOMEN'S EMPOWERED HEALING**

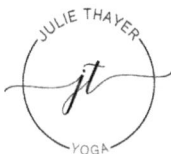

JULIE THAYER
jt
YOGA

JULIE THAYER

For Ollie, my love, my light.

*For the earth angels who carried me
when I could not carry myself.*

My gratitude is infinite.

It's time to celebrate!

Access Your Free RECLAIMED Library Here

As a way of saying thank you for purchasing a copy of my book, I am gifting you unlimited access to the RECLAIMED Library, an exclusive bonus for readers of *Reclaimed!*

From my courageous loving heart to your courageous loving heart, here is a collection of meditation and movement practices to support your journey into sustainable pain-free living.
Happy and kind exploring!

https://bit.ly/accesslibrary

Connect with Julie Thayer here at:

Website: **juliethayeryoga.com**
Facebook Page: **Julie Thayer Yoga**
Instagram: **@juliethayeryoga**
LinkedIn: **Julie Thayer**

Foreword

When Julie asked me to do the honor of writing this foreword, I had a small window of time available to do it. At first, I told her I'd take a look and see if I'd be able to get it done in the timeframe required. Once I got a spare moment and started, I found myself eager, inspired, and propelled to keep reading. At which point, I got back to Julie and said, "Absolutely, I'd love to write the foreword!"

The tone of this book is like sitting one-on-one with Julie and having safe, loving, warm and confidential conversation. Julie's words are a blend of compassionate consoler, motivational coach, and tour guide. Having traversed the tough emotional and mental terrain of her own life, she has successfully forged a path for us to follow. Her wit and brilliance are absolutely apparent. Most importantly, it's very clear that the information and guidance she doles out is hard-earned from her having done the work, including deep, gut wrenching, soul-searching, and self-examination. Not only will you find that this is a storybook and an autobiographical recounting of her incredible journey, *Reclaimed!* also provides teachings and therapeutic techniques, a *how-to* for you to transform yourself.

I had the pleasure and joy of meeting Julie when she arrived at our facilities as a student several years ago. Many of the tools that Julie shares in this book that she's found helpful in her process are yoga techniques that either I or my guest teachers have taught in our yoga therapy training program, and that are taught in other similar programs around the world. While these tools may seem simple on the surface, they are in fact extremely powerful.

My first experience into this new wellness world started in the fall of 1984 when I was desperately seeking a way out of the suicidal hell, I had created for myself. I needed a complete overhaul physically, mentally, emotionally, and spiritually. I discovered a healing path in holistic health, aka a macrobiotic diet and lifestyle. In addition to a plant-based whole foods diet and yoga-like movement practices, macrobiotic lifestyle promotes cultivating inner peace through meditation and self-reflection, fostering a positive perspective based on greeting the world with gratitude. After several years of eating this way, doing the daily practices, and seeing the world from this new perspective I discovered that my depression and suicidal tendencies had gradually vanished.

Deeper emotional work came later. This part was needed and important, but in hindsight I understand that I was not ready to do this until I had first built up a reserve of physical and spiritual strength, and confidence within myself. The confidence came through staying on the healing path and not cheating or sabotaging myself. I needed this base before I could tackle the hidden world of trauma, and some of the deeper more painful issues. We can only bite off what we are ready and emotionally equipped to chew. We need to feel safe and steady within ourselves first. We need to be on stable ground before we can look at parts of ourselves that might rock the boat.

The program that Julie came to attend was born from years of teaching macrobiotic cooking classes (since 1993), yoga classes (since 2000), and yoga teacher training programs (since 2002). I was inspired to create an advanced yoga therapy training program from the desire to share these therapeutic techniques with fellow yoga teachers and students interested in self-development. It was time to formally offer what had been dramatically transformative and life-changing for me, and hundreds of my clients. In 2009, this was a fledgling field in Canada and still, years later, it's relatively unknown.

These evidence-based, scientifically proven meditation and breathing practices have been renamed by the psychiatry/ psychotherapy world as *mindfulness practice.* Even though many of these practices are hundreds of years old from ancient yoga and yoga therapy texts, the rebranding made it more palatable for mainstream science.

The structural alignment techniques that Julie illuminates in her book come from John Friend, the original founder-creator of Anusara Yoga, which blends heart-felt themes with ground-breaking therapeutic alignment techniques called Universal Principles of Alignment. I studied with John from 2003 to 2011, attending many workshops in various cities in the United States and Canada and have seen firsthand how these techniques have completely transformed people in pain to completely pain-free in minutes. The alignment principles are based on biomechanics and the simple fact that the more our bodies are out of balance, the more stress we are under, and this affects us physically and on all levels. When we reduce our imbalances, we reduce our stress.

Julie clearly and insightfully reveals we are not only what we eat, we are what we think, do, and speak. As we go through the motions of replacing self-defeating activity with health promoting activity, we are transforming ourselves, one breath, one movement, one thought at a time. The techniques Julie teaches absolutely change us on the cellular level.

The raw, intelligent, heart-felt, deeply personal, and authentic exploration of Julie's experiences and self-healing will undoubtedly touch each of us. Julie's courage is contagious and invites, no, implores us to question our own state of heart and mind, and perhaps the need to go deeper, grow further?

Julie's words ring true and relevant because she digs down into the nitty gritty of how we all think and feel. She uncovers essential universal truths and lays them on the table in the most honest, vulnerable, relatable way imaginable. And she shows us that this is where we find our truth and our strength. Most importantly, she shows us how to transform our current state to a better state.

While we each have our own unique cross to bear, we can learn from each other, share the burden of pain together and, ultimately, be lifted up by one another. We can heal ourselves. The fact that you have this book in your hands means you are ready. You're in for a treat!

KAREN HEAVEN CLAFFEY
Founder-President
Heaven on Earth & Integrated Health -
Osteopathy, Yoga, Wellness
DOMP, CYT, E-RYT 500

Wellness is a function of our daily habits.

Unwellness is a function of our daily habits

It's up to us to choose kindly.

Preface

As I write this, I am wrapping up my week-long writing retreat, sequestered in cottage country, completing my first full draft of this book. In many ways the writing has been effortless, flowing out of me as if it were meant to be.

What I have come to realize these past few days, is that this has been a story in the making for fifty-plus years. All my heartache, grief, cries for help, and suicide attempts, over the course of my life, have led to this moment in time. Without them, this book would simply not be happening.

In the past four years, I have moved through my deepest healing, utilizing the tools acquired over my tumultuous lifetime to make the decision to choose living over dying, to care for myself, to stand up for myself as a woman, and to choose being there for my now 16-year-old son. There is clarity, peace, and capacity. There is integrity, authenticity, and resiliency. I feel it in every cell of my being.

As a woman who has experienced her share of trauma, and battled life-threatening depression, immobilizing anxiety, and chronic physical pain, I can sit here today and say, unequivocally, it has carved out my destiny. What was once debilitating now fuels my purpose and passion, my desire to show up and serve the world, to make my difference.

This book is written for women because, quite frankly, women experience the world differently. We wear many hats and try to wear them all perfectly. We love and nurture from our heart, often at its own expense. We have maternal instincts that focus on the health and well-being of all life. These characteristics are quelled by the world we live in, buried beneath paternalistic layers of what we have been told we *should* be and do. We tuck it all away for another day because we don't have the time, energy, or skill to deal with it, and because we are supposed to be fearless, strong, and infinite in our capacity. So, we throw on our masks and keep going... until WE CAN'T. We no longer have the ability to show up for ourselves, let alone others. It only makes sense then that our healing journey has its own unique road map.

If you can relate to this, then this book is for you, from my heart to yours. A combination of daily, doable yoga and self-care strategies, peppered with journal entries from my personal recovery, client case studies, and so much more. It's raw. It's real. It's transformational. I am so glad you are here.

Julie xo

Acknowledgements

Firstly, to Yoga. I am indebted to this ancient practice traced back to Northern India 5000 plus years ago. I acknowledge all that yoga encompasses, as well as the many teachers who have contributed to its evolution from generation to generation. Thank you for finding your way into my life.

To my teachers, who have so graciously and abundantly shared their knowledge with me and whose teachings resonated so profoundly. You transformed my understanding of the scope of Yoga to nourish life, to empower healing. Ganga White, Tracey Rich, Sven Holcomb, Todd Norian, Natasha Rizopoulos, Karen Claffey, Theresa Gagnon, Neil Pearson, Jnani Chapman, Antonio Sausys, Kristine Kaoverii Weber, Amy Weintraub, and Nitin Shah M.D. Ayu, your voices continue to guide me daily and I thank you from the bottom of my heart.

To my dear teacher, Karen Claffey, your mentorship has been invaluable to me in my journey as both a student and teacher of yoga. I am so very grateful for you. Thank you for lovingly crafting the foreword of my book. I am truly honored and my heart is full.

To my students, for whom I have had the honor of serving over the past ten years, you truly have been my greatest teachers, my greatest source of inspiration. As I always say, I feel I receive far more than I ever give. Much gratitude to you all.

To my fierce and fabulous book coach, Emma Hamlin, I could not have done this without your expert guidance, and your unrelenting love and support.

To my amazing editor, Kathy Olenski, thank you for kindly holding space for my words and helping me get it all just right!

To Danielle and Gerry Visco, so much gratitude for your friendship, and for sharing your sacred space so that I could retreat and write, undistracted and inspired.

To my hubby, who without fail captures moments. Photo credits for front and back cover belong to you, and I am most grateful. We are doing it, living the life we always wanted...cheers to us!

Last, but not least, to my cherished family and friends, thank you for walking with me and loving me through my journey.

Teamwork makes the dream work.

Introduction

I am often the last resort for my clients. They feel they have tried it all, bought the t-shirt. They are desperate for solutions to overcome physical, mental, and emotional pain, be it depression, anxiety, addiction, grief, body dysmorphia, or illnesses such as cancer, heart disease, autoimmune disease, Multiple Sclerosis (MS), Post Traumatic Stress Disorder (PSTD), Polycystic Ovary Syndrome (PCOS), and the list goes on. Together, we delve into the many facets of yoga to customize simple, effective strategies for whole health healing and recovery. And the best part? It's not rocket science but simple daily, doable practices that work.

Firstly, let me congratulate you for making this amazing decision for yourself. I am honored you are here to join me for this deep dive into the most important person in your life... YOU! You have chosen this book because you are ready to reclaim your life, to empower the healing of your mind, body, and soul, and to meet the ups and downs of your life with grace, capacity, and kindness.

What you also need to know is that this is a safe space. I have been where you are, I have also felt helpless and hopeless, my life ravaged by severe depression, anxiety, and suicide attempts. So, know this, "You are not alone. I see you, hear you, feel you, and celebrate you because I am you and you are me, and we are stronger together."

Speaking of safe space, the work I do with my clients is of a very deep and intimate nature and respecting the privacy of my clients is part of my professional oath. As such, all client reflections shared in this book are credited to participants of my RECLAIMED Mastery Program. Thank you for understanding the necessity for confidentiality, and for receiving the authenticity of their powerful words just the same. The inclusion of their experiences in this book is also a wonderful way for me to honor their transformational journeys.

Lastly, it would not be an exaggeration to say, yoga has contributed significantly to my life. Has it always been a love affair? Well, not exactly. I was an athlete in my younger years and, quite literally, my motto was "Harder. Stronger. Faster." Thus, my relationship with yoga was tenuous. Over the years, however, a nagging curiosity compelled me repeatedly back to my mat until eventually I began to embrace the idea that less is more. And then I fell hard and fast for this yoga thing, joyfully understanding that connection to breath, mindful movement, and kind alignment, supports the integration of the whole being. It inspires vitality in all the layers of one's being, physically, mentally, emotionally, energetically, and soulfully. This is the magic of yoga.

How has yoga changed my life specifically? I credit it for saving me from back surgery. I had been struggling with debilitating chronic pain, stemming from disc herniation in my lower back, and severe sciatica. After my initial consult with my surgeon, a surgeon whose preference was not to do surgery, I ceased all my other activities, but continued to nudge the edges of my physical discomfort with breath-work, mindfulness, and gentle yoga. When I saw the surgeon six weeks later, he said to me, "If you were one of my surgery patients in recovery, I would say you are progressing brilliantly! Keep doing what you are doing. No surgery." By my follow-up appointment, I had eased my pain and increased my range of motion so significantly, operating was not necessary. It has been ten pain-free years.

Where yoga has had the greatest impact upon the quality of my life, is relative to my mental health and, more specifically, inspiring the capacity to self-manage both depression and anxiety. The tools, or more accurately, the gifts of my personal, daily yoga practice have been infinite and made all the difference in my healing, recovery, and survival. And I want to share it all with you in this book. Why? So that you may show up for yourself, in any given moment, meeting the magic and mayhem of your beautiful life, physically, mentally, emotionally, energetically, and soulfully, with grace, resiliency, gratitude, and so much love.

What You Will Need:

- An open mind and an open heart
- A journal and a pen
- Yoga mat
- Yoga blocks (2)
- Blankets (2)
- Bolster (mid-size)
- Yoga strap

Gentle Reminders:

- Remember, this is YOUR EXPERIENCE. You know your breath, body, and mind best. Practice at your own pace... take a break when needed... absolutely use your props to support safe and spacious exploration. You are nudging edges here. Do this kindly, patiently, compassionately, and lovingly... no kicking doors down! Yoga should never feel painful in your physical body... ever!

- Emotional release is possible and may take various forms over the course of your journey, be it joy, sadness, worry, anger, frustration. Go slow... meet it... receive it... hold all the space necessary to move through it... again at your own pace. If it is bigger than what feels manageable for you, please reach out to me so that I am aware and may offer my support and guidance. I may also recommend reaching out to your healthcare professional for additional care, if needed.

Are you ready to reclaim your life with real, simple yogic tools? LET'S DO THIS!

Table of Contents

From Julie's Journal & Journey

They say a picture speaks
a thousand words
March 01st, 2018

…or does it? This picture was taken on November 30th, 2017, my birthday. I had just finished teaching class, truly one of my most joyful places to be, being of service and sharing yoga whilst being celebrated in the Birthday Chair amongst my dear friends and yoga community. I was smiling, laughing, and for all intents and purposes appeared to be having a blast. Darkness, however, was nipping at my heels. Inside, I was falling to pieces and, for the most part,

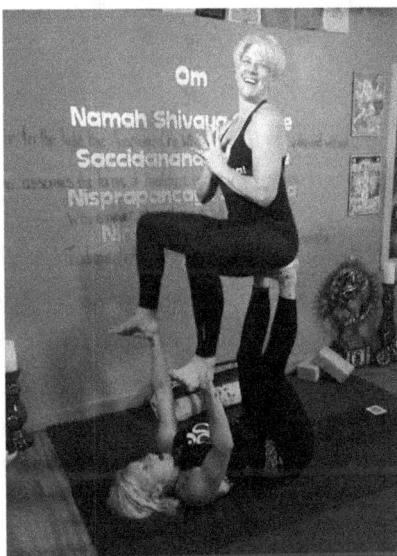

I was oblivious to the cataclysmic crash looming above me. After all, I had been managing my depression for many, many years, navigating the ups and downs of life with no problem! Whatever this was, I had it. But I didn't! Not eight hours later, I was being checked into the hospital, explaining to a Crisis Counsellor what had unfolded for me and why I was there. I was a shell of myself and remember saying, "Suddenly, there was only darkness, no light. I could not see any light... I always see the light." I recounted for him the events of the few months leading up to this day, and he referred to it as the perfect storm. In fact, he was right, it was. Hindsight is 20/20. If only I had been paying more attention, I may have felt the storm brewing and I may have been able to curtail its magnitude. Instead, I spent the next three weeks in the hospital trying to make rhyme or reason of how I arrived there, literally jaw on the floor.

Today, March 01st, 2018, marks 3 months. It has been a terrifying and wondrous ride... excruciating and extraordinary. Jam-packed with baby steps forward, setbacks, successes, stumbles, epiphanies, giant leaps forward, and massive growth. I distinctly remember having a conversation with my stepmom whilst I was in the hospital, and it became a defining moment for me. Her words: "Julie, you have a history of recovery and those who have a history of recovery, have a greater capacity to do so in the event of a relapse. You have beat this before, you will do it again." Her words inspired hope and possibility. I dug even deeper.

Later today I have a follow-up appointment with my psychiatrist. Yes, I have a psychiatrist, as part of my Mental Health Support Team. This team also includes nurses, a social worker, an occupational *therapist, and a counselor. My shrink (his word) and I are a good fit, and this is tremendously important in facilitating the healing process. He is, and has been, amazing and I am excited to check in with him. It has been well over a month since our last appointment, and I have oodles to share with him, relative to the work I have been doing and my ongoing recovery. Quite frankly, I think he is going to be a little blown away because honestly, I am. My stepmom was right, I can do this. I AM DOING IT. Every breath, every moment, every step I take, I feel myself regaining strength and confidence, and the best part, evolving into a more human, more real, more authentic version of me. And more than ever, I am determined to stay the path and explore, with wonder, what's next in my self-care journey and this crazy, magical thing called life. I wish the very same for you.*

IN THE CASE OF MENTAL HEALTH OR ADDICTIONS EMERGENCY/CRISIS:

If you, or someone you know, is experiencing a mental health or addiction crisis and requires emergency assistance, **CALL 911 or GO TO THE NEAREST HOSPITAL.**

CHAPTER 1

The Three Pillars of Pain-Free Living

Sustainable healing is built on an intentional, unshakeable foundation. Over the course of 20-plus years of experience, honing my movement and self-care expertise, I have identified what I call the *Three Pillars of Pain-Free Living* and they will serve as the touchstones for all that we explore together in this book.

Pillar One: AUTHENTIC AWARENESS

The practice of going gently inward and NOTICING... to kindly, authentically, explore and observe the breath, body, mind, energy, and soul... to gather insights... to graciously attend to sensation and experience. No judgment.

Pillar Two: COMPASSIONATE CONNECTION

The practice of intentional connection to sensation, emotion, and energy. Learning to sit in the experience, compassionately nudging the edges of unease, resistance, discomfort with an open mind and open heart.

Pillar Three: ALIGNED ACTION

Through daily, deeper awareness and connection, empowering mindful, purposeful action, such as breathwork, movement, mindfulness, and meditation practices, to impel yourself towards your optimal state of being, in any given moment... meeting the ups and downs of life with grace, capacity, and kindness.

We will return to these three pillars, over, and over, again, practicing the daily habit of utilizing the many doorways of yoga to bring clarity, tangibility, meaning, and functionality to these concepts.

THIS IS HEART-CENTERED, INTENTIONAL LIVING.

The 3 PILLARS OF PAIN-FREE LIVING

Making a daily habit of the many facets of yoga to bring clarity, tangibility, and meaning to these concepts. This is the practice.

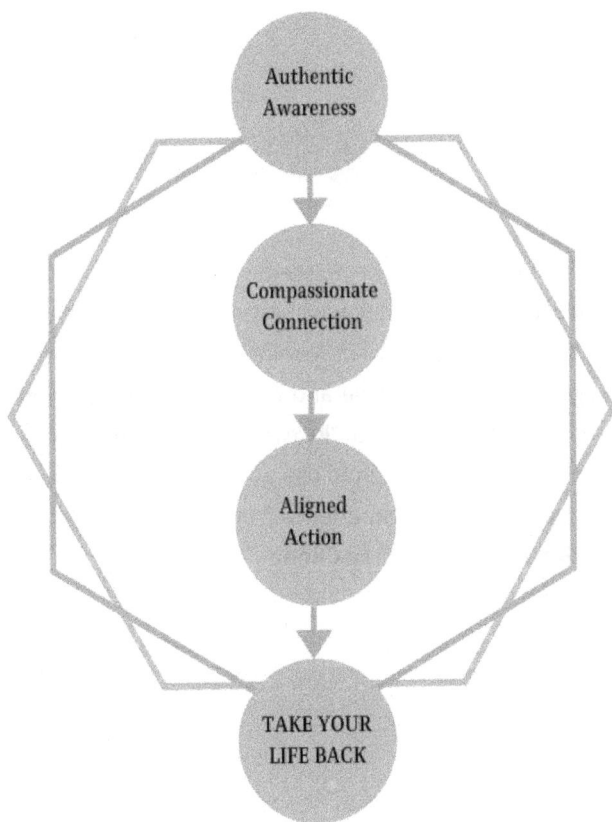

The magic is literally within you, and you are going to learn to access it to construct your infallible pillars.

ARE YOU READY?

"Julie's 3 Pillars of Pain-Free Living provides me with a trusted foundation to which I may return when my pain is knocking at the door. Reminding me to slow down, to go inward, to observe and connect to my experience, without judgement, to "love myself through" (as Julie so often says), and then to use the tools I have learned to steadily shift my experience from pain to peace."

- Reclaimed Mastery Client

From Julie's Journal & Journey

Learning to be and breathe in "THE GAP"
March 16th, 2018

To say that I received the greatest care imaginable during my hospital stay would be an understatement. From intake counselors, to nurses, to psychiatrists, to social workers, to occupational therapists, to fellow patients, I was cared for with kindness, compassion, non-judgement, and respect. The value in this alone, particularly when one is in such a vulnerable state of being, is of critical importance and sets the foundation for the journey of healing and recovery. Now I also needed to show up and do the work, relative to the myriad of resources offered to me and I will admit at times the work was beyond excruciating. For the first little while, it would have appeared I was getting my shit together. I got up early every day; did yoga for an hour or more; grabbed my coffee, once I had my off-ward privileges; ate brekkie, lunch, and dinner, even though I had no appetite; ran on the treadmill; participated in the vast majority of group sessions; met with my psychiatrist and nurses daily; interacted with and supported the other patients; walked the ward constantly, to keep moving; did more yoga in the afternoon; read oodles, and for all intents and purposes gave the appearance of improvement. There were very few tears and I really believed I was getting stronger every day. I was a 'model' patient.

Now, don't get me wrong, all the above was great self-care work but, and this is a really big BUT it was missing the boat on one very key aspect of my recovery, addressing my mental-emotional well-being. And I was in the mental health ward! It took a specific incident to make me aware of this gap in my thought process and behavior

As I mentioned earlier, I participated in virtually all the group sessions with one exception, music therapy. Music has the capacity to stir my soul deeply and crack my heart wide open. When I am in the throes of navigating depression, my greatest fear is my heart doing just that. When my feelings are so incredibly overwhelming, I believe I may not survive them. Hence, I avoid music with everything I have got! One evening I was asked to join the music therapy group. Firstly, there was acoustic guitar, which is definitely a no-go for me, and secondly, it was in a small room jammed with people and the claustrophobic me was also digging in her heels as well. I politely declined, stating that, "Unless it's going to be hard core rock and put a skip in my step, I'm out." The facilitator tried to entice me, saying that there would be all styles of music, including rock, but I resisted, "Nope, not doing it." I did agree to a compromise i.e., walking the hallway so that I could listen from afar. At the first twang of the guitar, I felt the tears begin to stir and by the end of my first lap the tears were streaming. I did, however, keep walking.

Now earlier that day, I also had my second session with my occupational therapist (OT), who had been introducing me to a form of therapy called Dialectal Behavior Therapy (DBT). We were doing some very good work together and the focus in that particular session was on Self-Awareness. I was given homework, completed it brilliantly, of course, as again I was a model patient. In fact, I had created this beautiful circle graph, very colorful and pretty, depicting the various events that precipitated The Perfect Storm and my consequent segue into the darkness.

My third session with my OT was the very next day, on the coat-tails of my music therapy extravaganza. My psychiatrist joined us for the first part of the session. I explained to them both what had unfolded for me whilst participating indirectly in group the previous night. I explained the music did me in and resulted in my walking and crying up and down the halls. My psychiatrist then said to my OT, "Do you hear that? There is the event that elicits the response, in this case, the crying, but no explanation of what the feelings are that go with it. There is a gap here."

My OT nodded in agreement. I was asked what I was feeling when listening to the music and I thought about it, really hard I might add, but I had nothing. Busted! I remember my psychiatrist sighing vehemently and then saying, "This is why you are seeing a shrink!" At which point he got up and left. Enter the Tough Love. The session continued and I proudly presented my homework. My OT studied it with great attentiveness and asked me some pointed questions, which I dug very deep to answer and which inevitably resulted in kicking open the floodgates.

She looked at me with great compassion and said, "Julie, you have done a really good job putting your thoughts to paper here. Having reviewed it I would like to suggest that a great deal of what you are choosing not to face, or feel, is grief. Do you think that is possible?" And well, that was the tipping point. At the word grief, I let go physically, mentally, emotionally... the sobbing literally wracking my body... grief exploding my brain. My OT simply held the space for me to surrender to it all... no judgement, simply presence, patience, and a whole lot of genuine care. I had been in the hospital for almost three weeks, and it was the first time I had given myself permission to sit with, and feel, every agonizing, gutting loss. It was a significant leap in my healing, as I discovered that I could hang out in THE GAP and survive. I learned later there had been a supportive celebration between my OT and nurses, as they had all been awaiting my breaking down of the fortress in which I had sequestered myself. What a wonderful thing to have cheerleaders!

Over three months later, more time spent playing in THE GAP, more learning, more progress, more healing. Is it still hard? Yes. I still have some pretty down moments, even days. What's the difference? I am managing the difficult emotions more effectively and they are no longer lingering or asserting themselves to the same degree as in the acute stages of my depression. So, yes, it is getting easier. Am I grateful? Am I hopeful? Excited about the future? Do I dare to dream? A big, beautiful YES to all that and then some. I am getting so much better at sitting authentically in the tough stuff, facing it, and feeling it in real time, so that years later it doesn't come back to bite me in the ass! I am also *celebrating what a gift it is to feel and to experience this life so deeply, with healthy boundaries to boot. This is the magic of full throttle living. I am feeling more freedom in all aspects of my being and becoming more me than I've ever been.*

CHAPTER 2

Make Your Whole Health Your First Priority

Choose yourself today for healthier
and happier tomorrows.

Yep, from this day forward, you are just going to do it. Every single day. And yes, ahead of your kids, your partner, your employer, your dog, your cat, the laundry, and the house cleaning. When you begin to perceive and accept yourself as a whole being, you amplify your capacity for healing. When you choose to show up for yourself, first and foremost, you may then show up for the rest of your life, as the very best possible version of you, physically, mentally, emotionally, energetically, and soulfully. This is not selfishness. This is smart self-care. This is yoga.

Ways you can make this happen for yourself:

- **Make your mornings count**. I can't emphasize this enough. There is time to be found in the morning, before the rest of the household and world wakes, before you are required to be present and 'on,' when the likelihood of you committing to a regular self-care routine is so much greater. The more you delay it and think "It's ok, I will get to it later." the more undoable and elusive it becomes. Why? Because life happens and you get pulled in a gazillion directions. By the time you circle back to yourself, you are starving, physically exhausted, and mentally done in. And surprise, you find yourself knee-deep in the mindless *Eat-Do-Sleep-Repeat Cycle*. Am I right?

Reflect upon your morning routine. Work back from your first commitment in the day. What time are you required to really show up in your day? What time do you currently wake to ensure you are ready to meet it? Can you wake up 5 minutes earlier? 15? 30? 60? According to a recent study by University of Colorado Boulder, waking just one-hour earlier cuts depression risk by 23 per cent.[1] I, myself, rise at 4:45 a.m. every day, for the sole purpose of practicing self-care. What does this look like? Keep in mind, I have been at this for a while now, so I am highly disciplined at making it happen easily. It includes 30-75 minutes of yoga, (a combination of breath, kind movement, mindfulness, and meditation), and walking briskly for one hour, five mornings per week. I invest, at most, 135 minutes per day, in intentional self-care. This equates to 9.38% of a 24-hour day, less than ten percent! I am worth this...and so are you!

If you are currently making magic with your mornings, amazing, keep it up! If there is an opportunity for you to capture more of your day and make it productive, I encourage you to practice doing just that. Literally, set

---

1   Science Daily, "Waking just one-hour earlier cuts depression risk by double digits, study finds." https://www.sciencedaily.com/releases/2021/05/210528114107.htm, Source: The University of Colorado Boulder, May 28, 2021

your alarm and do it. It won't necessarily feel easy in the beginning, but I guarantee you once you inspire the habit, you will have more energy, greater clarity, and purpose, as you navigate the remainder of your day. And the contents of this book are going to provide you with a smorgasbord of simple tools, to ensure you are making the most of your precious, new-found gift of time! Moreover, you are also going to learn how to create *islands of calm* in your day. Seamless, actionable moments of breath, mindfulness, and movement, here, there, and everywhere, so that you remain in the driver's seat of your best self.

- **Nourishing Nights.** It was a client who, so astutely, pointed out to me, that the success of her morning routine is directly influenced by the efficacy of her night routine. The fact is, how you choose to manage both your mornings and nights matters significantly. They are inextricably linked. A consistent, mindful wind-down, each evening, is imperative. 'Resting' is just as important as the 'Doing.'

Here are some ways to inspire nourished nights:

1. **Intentional Technology Time-Out.** Decide on a realistic time to come off your technology, particularly your phone, to rest your eyes and your brain, and to curtail the pressure to respond. Allow this action to signify that the '*on demand*' part of your day is done.

2. **Hold space for quality quiet time.** Conversation, journaling, reading, bathing, meditating, to name but a few. Invite an intentional slow down over the course of your evening.

3. **TV and technology out of the bedroom.** Hold space for minimal distraction and optimal rest.

4. **7-9 hours remains the magic window for most adults[2].** Obviously, there will be exceptions but, as consistently as possible, make this a priority. Just as your muscles need time to repair after a workout, so does your mind and body after the day-to-day demands of active life. To the best of your ability, aim to go to bed at the same time each night. Create a routine. Sleep can be one of your most powerful allies when it comes to living your best life.

> *Sleep and watchfulness, when*
> *immoderate, constitute disease.*
> *- Hippocrates*

TRANSFORMATIONAL INSIGHT: Traditionally, we think of Yoga as arriving upon our mat for a scheduled class, to breathe and to move our bodies. But, in fact, the practice begins the moment we wake up, that first moment we return our conscious awareness to that first sip of air, to physical sensation, mood, emotions, and energy. Taking time to nudge edges... a little stretch here, a little stretch there... gathering insights as to the state of our being in that moment... embracing our aliveness, celebrating it.

The Yoga then continues throughout the day, in varying degrees of effectiveness, depending upon our capacity to attend to present moment, to be aware, to connect.

---

2   National Institute of Neurological Disorders and Stroke, "Brain Basics: Understanding Sleep", National Institutes of Health, https://www.ninds.nih.gov/Disorders/Patient-Caregiver-Education/Understanding-Sleep, Published August 13, 2019

From this deeper place of connection, we inspire mindful, purposeful, action. And, in the process, propel ourselves forward, toward our optimal state of being.

This is the daily practice, the moment-to-moment exploration of our experience, physically, mentally-emotionally, energetically, and soulfully.

- **Write your story**. Your story matters. When I was in the hospital recovering from my suicide attempt in November of 2017, my psychiatrist suggested that I begin a journal, a seemingly innocuous request. Except, I am an introvert and extracting the thoughts swirling about in my head, making sense of them, and getting them to land on paper was nothing short of excruciating. My first attempts, in my opinion, were abysmal and resulted in pages being ripped out, torn to bits, and dismissively tossed in the trash. My doctor gently encouraged me to keep going... to ditch the self-judgement and my need for it to be some sort of literary masterpiece... to simply keep writing. So, I did. And let me tell you, the dam broke. The words, they began flowing and they haven't stopped since.

   Writing has been instrumental to my healing and recovery, and, if it is not something you currently practice, I would encourage you to start. This is your opportunity to connect more deeply with your inner world, to process your thoughts, and feelings... to chart your progress... to get it out.

Perhaps you begin by taking 5-10 minutes of your morning self-care routine to set intentions for the day, to write them out, to visualize them. And in the evening, you take another 5-10 minutes to reflect upon your day, good, bad, ugly, and/or indifferent. No expectations, no pressure. Wish to write more? Do it. Less? Do it. But DO IT. Daily. Even five minutes can yield a profound return on investment. Yours is a story of empowered healing and it deserves to be told, not only for your benefit, but perhaps, when the time is right, you may be of service to others.

> *One day you will tell your story of how you overcame what you went through, and it will be someone else's survival guide.*
> *- Brené Brown*

- **Making Space**: Create your own Whole Health Nook, a special place to settle fully into self-exploration, breath, meditation, and movement. And before you get crazy, thinking renovation budget and what room you will convert (the second bathroom-ha! ha!), take a deep breath and scale it back, sister! You are going for simplicity here. What I am suggesting is finding a place, maybe it's the corner of your bedroom, big enough for your yoga mat and props. Perhaps a little table, where you might place a few of your favorite things, books, trinkets, affirmation cards, candles, artwork... your child's Grade 1 ceramic coaster project, for instance! Items for which you feel a deep affinity and connection, that spark, at first sight, a feeling of goodness within you. In yoga, this is often referred to as an altar. What it really is, is a sacred, safe place, meant just for you, nobody else...not the kids, the partner, the dog, the cat, just you.

Have fun with this *little* project, emphasis on the word little. Note, this should not take you hours... thirty minutes, tops! Let your intuition guide you in your choice of space and treasures. Get creative. Remember, this nook is going to be part of your daily practice in self-care, so it will play a key role in your healing and recovery. We will discuss exactly how to do this when we talk about *Becoming Besties with Your Nervous System*.

- **Conversations with Yourself, About Yourself**

Consciously choose to rise up and into your worth, to the very best of your ability, in any given moment. Especially in those tougher moments, when your unrelenting, misguided inner voice is revving up turbo-style and fiercely determined to convince you otherwise. Dig deep... silence that voice... shift the dialogue... to one of kindness, acceptance, patience, and love.

OK, so I am going to share a story here. One morning, post-suicide attempt, I decided to practice some yoga. I literally had to force myself to get on my mat. My mind, heart, and body felt heavy, and I could feel the tears percolating and eventually becoming a torrential downpour. One of the things I was working on, was giving myself permission to cry, to face and process the feelings I feared the most. I also read somewhere, that tears from a really good cry were as beneficial as a spa facial. So, YAY, it was going to be a win-win! So, that day, despite the steady stream, I kept breathing, kept moving, and kept exploring the darker parts of myself, which eventually had me examining the conversation I was having with myself, about myself.

Going to backtrack a bit here. When I found myself in crisis back in November 2017, I had envisioned myself wearing this t-shirt. To clarify, I don't actually own this t-shirt and I do hope it is not available for purchase anywhere. But in my mind, it was what I saw. I felt it summed me up in a nutshell. From a girl celebrated for her *pink-colored-glasses* approach to life, talk about a shocking admission. Somewhere along the line, I had started being very unkind to myself and, even worse, somewhere along the line, I had let it become my truth. I had been sucked into what I now officially refer to as *The Vortex*.

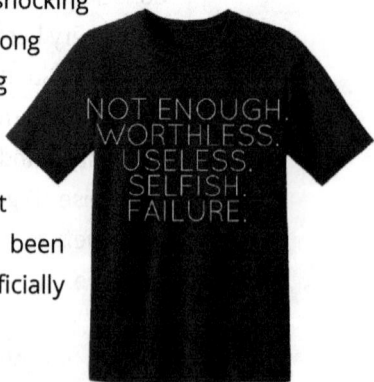

NOT ENOUGH.
WORTHLESS.
USELESS.
SELFISH.
FAILURE.

The not-so-good thing about that morning practice was, that I found myself hanging out in this Vortex. The oh-so-good part was, I caught myself before it swallowed me up. This was PROGRESS!

A note before I go any further… on the flip side, having positive, constructive, authentic inner dialogue does not mean abdicating responsibility, particularly if one's actions and decisions have resulted in the hurting of others. Have I made mistakes? YES. Have I hurt people I love? YES. Have I failed? YES. But have I learned? YES. Have I said sorry and meant it? YES. Have I pulled up my socks, tried again and experienced success? YES. Owning the good, the bad, and the ugly of my choices, balanced with the understanding that I am a perfectly imperfect human being doing the best I can with the information available to me is fundamental to my self-care and movement forward. I need to be as fair to myself, as I would be to another human being.

Do you have a t-shirt like the one above, with similar or somewhat different words? Do you consciously or unconsciously throw it on when life gets tough and is biting you in the ass? Now, let me ask you, if your best friend was struggling and came to you for support, would you gift them this t-shirt and say good luck with that? Of course not. In fact, the idea of doing so is preposterous, right? I know exactly how I would choose to respond to a friend or loved one in need. I would hold space, oodles of it. I would be honest, compassionate, patient, and non-judgmental in my words. I would remind her of her *more-than-enoughness*. I would gift her this white t-shirt, with a big-ass red bow, and tell her, "You've got this." And so, that morning, I gave myself just that and found myself lovingly, fearlessly fighting my way out of *The Vortex* and into the light.

So, right here, right now, I am gifting you this white t-shirt, with a big-ass red bow. I wish you to know I am here, I have your back, and I believe in you. This is also your gentle reminder to catch yourself, the moment your inner dialogue shifts to one of self-deprecation. This is your invitation to practice breaking the cycle... to be kind, compassionate, and patient... to love yourself, every damn day, like you would your most cherished friend.

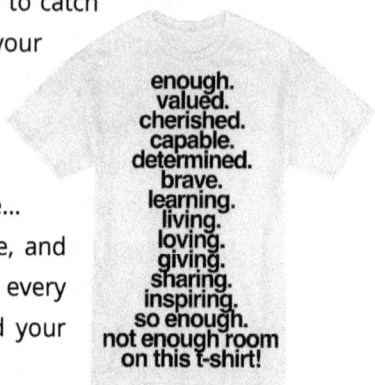

enough.
valued.
cherished.
capable.
determined.
brave.
learning.
living.
loving.
giving.
sharing.
inspiring.
so enough.
not enough room
on this t-shirt!

TO RECAP:

✓ You are learning to make your mornings count.

✓ You are learning the value of nourished nights.

✓ You are learning the value of writing your story of resilience and recovery.

✓ You are learning the value of creating a safe and sacred place for practice.

✓ You are learning the value of speaking to yourself with compassion and love.

✓ You are learning the value of honing awareness, deepening connection, and taking mindful, purposeful action.

✓ YOU ARE LEARNING TO MAKE A DAILY HABIT OF WELLNESS.

Are you ready to dive into the nitty-gritty? Beginning with a discussion in **Chapter 3: Becoming Besties with Your Nervous System**. Yes! For real!

"I realize how often I resort to negative self-talk, and what a habit it has become for me. Now all I hear is Julie's voice in my head, 'Talk to yourself like you are the love of your life: YOU ARE.' As a result, I am getting better and better at catching myself earlier in the conversation and shifting to an inner dialogue that is honest, supportive, and loving. I find I am celebrating myself more and more every day and this feels really good."

-1:1 RECLAIMED Mastery Client

From Julie's Journal & Journey

Falling into the ebb and flow of change
March 25th, 2018

"Nothing ever comes to rest. Everything keeps moving. Even stationary objects are moving, though we do not see it. Change is constant and that means we are not the same from one moment to another either. Our cells are constantly in the process of changing. So, if I am moving through a tough situation, there is no point trying to find "rest" so that I can cope. That is impossible. Instead, I can choose to change trajectory, to move in a direction that will lead me toward peace. THAT is always attainable."

- Richard Wagamese, Embers

In a week's time I will be in the throes of moving day and diving headfirst into more change. A positive and necessary step, only eleven kilometers away, and it brings me just a little closer to living on a larger water body. YAY for me and my SUP board! Yet today my anxiety is percolating. Symptoms include heart palpitations, shortness of breath, the left side of my chest feeling like it is being squeezed in a vice, and my body spontaneously shaking. No fun. I therefore have spent my day practicing lots of intentional self-care, slowing it all down with connection to breath, mindful movement on my yoga mat and kind, compassionate inner dialogue. Grateful.

As Richard Wagamese says, change is a constant. For many years I was the 'master of change,' to the point I would get excited and embrace the possibilities that ebbed and flowed with its uncertainty. I trusted in the silver linings that inevitably presented themselves and I believed somehow it was all going to be OK. When life imploded for me last fall, I found myself sideswiped by colossal change. I also found myself completely unprepared to meet the challenges I had created for myself... you heard me right... created for myself. It is easy to think of change as 'happening' to us. However, we cultivate change through even our teeniest-tiniest choices and actions. I made many decisions, some great ones and some I wish I had made differently, decisions that became the catalyst for the spectacular shift in my life. I willingly own them all. And, yes, there were certain things beyond my control, choices made by others and circumstances, but even in this regard I had a choice as to how I responded, as in gracefully or not. Let's just say the grace part eluded me a few times! In the aftermath of my crisis, I felt like I needed to fix everything all at once. Decisions and amends needed to be made and I put tremendous pressure upon myself to do just that. Suffice it to say it was crushing me and very unhelpful in my healing and recovery. Thankfully, a couple of my support peeps kindly reminded me, "Julie, you do not need to make all of these decisions NOW. In fact, now is probably not a good time at all. You are raw, healing, and recovering, not exactly a place from which good decision-making springs. Give yourself space, take one decision at a time, and move forward in baby steps."

I took that one step further, making them 'baby-toe' steps: forward movement, nonetheless, and enough.

I feel I have accomplished only twenty percent of the work, relative to all the above, and that in the last couple of months I have simply been laying the foundation for the remaining eighty percent... Pareto's Principle at its best! A little daunting, yes, and likely the impetus for today's anxiety. What I do know is, in this decision to move, I am making an active, conscious choice in the trajectory of my life, and I also trust that it is leading me towards greater peace and possibility. The reality is I was seeking change, facilitating it, and thus I am exactly where I am meant to be, on the path I created for myself. Depression and anxiety aside, I cannot complain or be disappointed in the chaos and crisis that ensued. I chose it and so must embrace it... breaking down to break through. I will continue to practice self-care, diligently, but I will not rest. One baby-toe step at a time in all the directions that compel me toward greater ease, and a simpler, more spacious, inspired-life. Deep breath in, deeper breath out.

CHAPTER 3

Becoming Besties with Your Nervous System

I would be remiss if I did not take time to talk about the nervous system and how yoga can support a healthy balance between the sympathetic nervous system (fight-flight-freeze-fawn) and the parasympathetic nervous system (rest-digest-rejuvenate). Too many human beings in the First World are walking around with a nervous system in overdrive. In the United States, from 2014 – 2019, the value of the prescribed drugs market for nervous system disorders, grew from almost $15 billion to $20 billion U.S. dollars, making this one of the top therapeutic needs in the United States[3]. It is really the new norm of function... do more... strive more... do it in less time... use fewer resources... regardless of boundaries. Left unattended, this is making us sick, physically, mentally, and, in some cases, killing us. These are verifiable facts.

Yoga, inclusive of asana (movement), pranayama (controlled breath), meditation, and mindfulness, is, thank goodness, a powerful moderator of the nervous system. Think of it this way.

---

3   Matej Mikulic, "Value of U.S. nervous system disorders from 2014 to 2019", Statista, Health, Pharma & Medtech, Pharmaceutical Products & Market, https://www.statista. com/statistics/445671/us-nervous-system-disorders-market-size/, Published September 20, 2021

Your yoga practice has the capacity to turn the volume DOWN, not off, on your over-effective fight-flight-freeze-fawn response and turn the volume UP on your much over-muscled, under-utilized rest-digest-rejuvenate system. It is in this shift that balance is restored, and healing and recovery become possible.

This is huge. Why? Because you just discovered that all that you need is within you. Take a deep, beautiful breath in and receive this empowering insight. You, yourself, have the capacity to influence the state of your nervous system.

TRANSFORMATIONAL INSIGHT: To heal effectively and sustainably, we must first feel safe.

This is the reason creating your Whole Health Nook is so important. Your brain and nervous system recognize it as a safe space where you can show up, just as you are, for kind exploration and self-care.

OK, story time! This one is titled *"Anxiety, a Hostile Takeover."* Firstly, I wish to discuss the stats relative to anxiety in Canada, where I live.

According to Statistics Canada: One in ten Canadians will have at least one anxiety disorder in their lifetime.[4]

---

4   Government of Canada, "Mental-Health Anxiety Disorders", https://www.canada.ca/en/health-canada/services/healthy-living/your-health/diseases/mental-health-anxiety-disorders.html, Published July 2009

Mood Disorders Society of Canada describes Anxiety Disorders as, "Intense and prolonged feelings of fear and distress that occur out of proportion to the actual threat or danger. The feelings of fear and distress interfere with normal daily functioning."[5]

We are going to focus upon Generalized Anxiety Disorder (GAD). The MAYO Clinic defines Generalized Anxiety Disorder as "Excessive anxiety and worry about a number of events or activities occurring for more days than not over a period of at least six months with associated symptoms, such as fatigue and poor concentration." The Mayo Clinic goes on to describe the symptoms of GAD as follows:

Generalized Anxiety Disorder symptoms can vary. They may include:

- Persistent worrying or anxiety about a number of areas that are out of proportion to the impact of the events
- Overthinking plans and solutions to all possible worst-case outcomes
- Perceiving situations and events as threatening, even when they aren't
- Difficulty handling uncertainty
- Indecisiveness and fear of making the wrong decision
- Inability to set aside or let go of a worry
- Inability to relax, feeling restless, and feeling keyed up or on edge

5   Mood Disorders Society of Canada, "The Human Face of Mental Health and Mental Illness in Canada". Chapter 5 - Anxiety Disorders, 80, http://mdsc.ca/documents/ Consumer%20and%20Family%20Support/Anxiety%20disorders_EN.pdf

- Difficulty concentrating, or the feeling that your mind "goes blank"

Physical signs and symptoms may include:

- Fatigue

- Trouble sleeping

- Muscle tension or muscle aches

- Trembling, feeling twitchy

- Nervousness or being easily startled

- Sweating

- Nausea, diarrhea, or irritable bowel syndrome

- Irritability

The Mayo Clinic continues to explain, "There may be times when your worries don't completely consume you, but you still feel anxious even when there's no apparent reason. For example, you may feel intense worry about your safety or that of your loved ones, or you may have a general sense that something bad is about to happen."[6]

---

6   The Mayo Clinic, Anxiety Disorders, Patient Care & Health Information, Diseases & Conditions, https://www.mayoclinic.org/diseases-conditions/anxiety/symptoms-causes/syc-20350961

In my past, I struggled solely with depression and thus, with many years of counselling and the creation of a toolkit to help me proactively manage my symptomology, depression, in essence, became *The Devil I Knew*. Anxiety, not so much. With the arrival of *The Perfect Storm* in September of 2017, and my subsequent suicide attempt in November of 2017, anxiety had clearly decided it was missing out and would love to join the party! Enter the hostile takeover... heart palpitations, difficulty breathing, spontaneous body tremors, nausea, overwhelming exhaustion, and complete immobilization. All seemingly out of the blue and beyond my control. In a word, brutal. Especially when I'm to be on my mat to lead a yoga class in less than thirty minutes. Where am I? Pulled over on the side of the road, shaking uncontrollably, head between knees, heaving cookies, full on basket-case, and thinking, how in the Bleep! Bleep! Bleep! am I going to do this... which by the way, only served to exacerbate all the above to the nth degree.

For me, I experience anxiety as a *whole-being invasion*, a possession, in fact, with the line, "Exorcise the Demons," singing gleefully in my head. Maybe you can relate?

Fortunately, through yoga and my understanding of the nervous system, I gained clarity on the impetus for my anxiety. During my self-implosion of 2017, I experienced several traumas simultaneously, one after the other, some, my own doing, others inspired by external influences, and simply beyond my control. They hit hard, fast, and mercilessly, cranking the volume up on my sympathetic nervous system... you know the good ol' fight-flight-freeze-fawn response until I realized I was moving through my recovery efforts waiting for the other shoe to drop... for the next trauma to sucker-punch me, and lucky me, with a nervous system more determined than ever to keep me safe from the big bad, world. With this epiphany, I also knew exactly what needed to be done. Any guesses? Yeah, you got it, I turned to my tried-and-true lifesaver yoga… or what I playfully refer to as my *superpower*.

One day, early in my recovery, I was reflecting on things from a yoga perspective. I realized I had moved through significant, simultaneous, multiple traumas, some within my control and some beyond, and my sympathetic nervous system, as it does in situations like this went into turbo-mode to protect me from further trauma, to keep me safe. In essence, even though I was moving forward with counselling and working towards recovery, my brain and nervous system had other plans. They were in a perpetual state of waiting for the next trauma to hit. When I recognized this, I was able to hold space for myself with a greater degree of patience and compassion. I began to approach my healing differently and I sought a more restorative form of yoga practice. By slowing things down, settling into breath, mindfulness, and meditation, I was literally, over time, able to change the story being relayed between my brain and nervous system. My brain finally got on board with the fact that I was no longer in imminent danger and kindly communicated to my over-zealous nervous system… "She's OK. She's safe. We're safe." Today, my yoga practice helps to keep my anxiety at bay, it helps me cope with the symptoms and manage myself proactively. Does this make sense? This is the magic of a consistent yoga practice…the profound potency of breath, movement, mindfulness, and meditation.

What's the takeaway here? The moment we feel that first strained breath, that first overzealous beat of our heart, that first hint of a tremor beneath our skin, we have the power within us to take control, to change the trajectory of our anxiety. Does this alone, not have you feeling hope? With practice, we can change our story, and this is damn exciting. My true desire with this book, is to bring a deeper understanding of the capacity we have within ourselves to take charge of our experience, to change our story. Breath, kind movement, and mindfulness can inspire a different experience in us, one of empowerment, hope and healing!

So, guess what? You are going to become besties with your nervous system. Firstly, by simply practicing a keen awareness of its presence, function, and impact upon your state of being. You are going to attend to it daily, as you would a garden, pulling weeds, and nourishing it with intentional breath, kind movement, and loving thoughts. And from this deeper connection, you will inspire mindful, purposeful action, igniting a much-needed recalibration of your nervous system.

TO RECAP:

✓ You now have a better understanding of the function of your nervous system and its impact on your state of being.

✓ You have also learned that yoga is a powerful moderator of the nervous system, which means, with practice, you have the capacity within you to recalibrate yourself; to heal and recover.

✓ You are going to befriend your nervous system, practicing daily, gentle awareness, attending to physical and mental-emotional sensation, connecting more deeply to your experience, so that you may inspire mindful, purposeful action toward your optimal state of being.

✓ YOU ARE LEARNING TO MAKE A DAILY HABIT OF BEING BESTIES WITH YOUR NERVOUS SYSTEM.

Now, I hear you saying, "Awesome, Julie, this sounds really, really great! But where the heck do I start?" Oh! How I love this question! As with most things, the best place is at the beginning. In the case of yoga, it always begins and ends with the breath.

And how convenient, this provides the perfect segue into **Chapter 4: Your Breath is The Bomb!** Here, we are going to talk the magic of the breath and specific techniques for managing all recoveries.

"Understanding the function of the nervous system, as it relates to my experience of pain, has been very enlightening. With this newfound knowledge, I am making a habit of self-care and making kinder choices, so that my nervous system feels supported and balanced. Overall, I am feeling more relaxed and more capable of managing my pain. It really has been a game-changer."

- RECLAIMED Mastery Client

From Julie's Journal & Journey

Sunshine, blue skies, fresh air, healing, and recovery
April 22nd, 2018

When the sun shines and blue skies prevail, I am irresistibly compelled to breathe and be outside. And being that the water temp is still on the chilly side for a date with my stand-up paddleboard I opted for a walk in my new neighborhood. Everybody was out and about, walking, running, biking, playing, driving with windows wide open, hanging out on patios, motorcycles galore, and smiles in abundance! You could almost hear the collective sigh as the weight of winter lifted off my shoulders… PURE JOY.

Back in late December, when I returned home from the hospital, I made a point of walking as often as I could, meaning pretty much daily, despite the weather. Everything about it felt hard. My mind and body were heavy, and there were often tears. From the beginning to the end, and with each step, I recited the mantra, "Healing, recovery, healing recovery, healing, recovery…" It felt like an effort in survival. However, moving vigorously, surrounded by nature, breathing in the fresh air, absorbing the Vitamin D, the days turned into weeks and the weeks turned into months, and I could literally feel the slow, steady healing of my mind, body, and soul. Today recovery feels real, and I feel more like myself than ever... each layer gently peeled back and a more authentic me revealed. Is it scary? Yes. Inspiring and exciting? Bigger YES! The best part is, I like her. I like the me I am becoming.

So, today, when I walked, there was no heaviness, but rather a sense of lightness and optimism. There was no need for mantra, my mind was attentive to the energy surrounding me. I could look around at the hustle and bustle, the aliveness of it all, feeling happy and hopeful. When I walked by the water, I dreamed of the warmer days ahead, floating on my SUP board, big blue skies above, soaking in the sunshine. Yes, life has changed in a big way, but I have the summer ahead to settle into a new home, routines, and community, and I believe it is going to be amazing. I also believe the following statement with my whole heart, "Recovery from depression and anxiety is possible with attentiveness to breath, mindfulness, kind movement, baby-toe steps, compassion, patience, and a whole lotta love... not just surviving but thriving."

I wish this for myself, I wish this for you. Why? That's easy. We are worth it.

CHAPTER 4

Your Breath is The Bomb!

Breathe. It may be all you can manage,
in this moment, and it is enough.

Breathing, no surprise, is important. When it comes to yoga, it is the most important. I have often said to my students, "If we simply came together on our mats, to breathe mindfully, the benefits would be more than enough to inspire transformation in all the layers of our being." Now, Pranayama takes breathing a step further, in that it is a means by which we intentionally affect change to the breath to support a desired outcome. A good example is Extended Exhalation, where the exhalation is purposely longer than the inhalation. You may breathe in for a count of 4 and exhale for a count of 6. This breath has been proven to be a very healing breath, in that it allows for greater release of toxins and invites a sense of calm to both the body and the mind. On the flip side, Ujjayi breath, also known as fire breath, builds heat and energy. Then there is Breath of Joy and it elicits, just that, joy! Nadi Shodhana, Alternate Nostril Breathing, brings balance to the right and left sides of the brain and body.

As you embark upon your yogic journey, you will come to learn there is an abundance of breathing techniques from which you may choose, and those that resonate with you may be added to your self-care toolkit, available to you anytime you may need them. Yoga at your fingertips, 24-7.

Now, let's explore some specific pranayamas.

THREE PART BREATH

1. Breathe in through your nose. Feel the coolness of the air as it passes in through your nostrils.

2. Draw the inhale fully into your belly (part 1), your rib cage (part 2), your chest (part 3), inviting expansion and space.

3. Now, release the breath fully in exhalation.

    - from your belly (part 1)

    - your rib cage (part 2)

    - your chest (part 3)

4. Feel its warmth as it passes through the nostrils.

5. Let go.

This is transformation in its simplest most organic form... from inhale to exhale... from fullness to emptiness... from coolness to warmth... from oxygen to carbon dioxide... from nourishment to waste. All this to maintain stability and equilibrium of our physiological processes. Many factors such as diet, hydration, exercise, alcohol, smoking, and stress levels affect how hard the body must work to support an optimal state of being. If balance cannot be restored and/or sustained, the body eventually says, "Enough!" and unattended vulnerabilities may eventually present themselves in the form of serious illness and disease.

Our mental health is no different. The fact is, like our bodies, our minds are hard-wired for change, adaptation, and evolution. Our capacity to think, reason, choose, and make decisions permits us to experiment, explore, and experience life in all its glory. We are by nature facilitators of change which sometimes serves us well, and sometimes does not. If we go too far down the path of self-neglect or even of self-destructive thoughts and behaviors, vulnerabilities may present themselves in the form of panic, anxiety, depression, and other mental health challenges. We then find ourselves battling fiercely to return to a state of stability and equilibrium.

Practicing diligent self-awareness, self-acceptance, and self-care is key to managing the ebb and flow of life. Change, welcome or not, is inevitable and if we choose to meet it with kindness, compassion, and patience, then we learn, grow, and transform. We live inspired.

ONE MINUTE SELF-CARE RESET

On average, adult humans take 12-18 breaths per minute. Need a timeout? Give yourself a *mindful minute* to simply breathe. If doable, take it outside for a bonus fresh air infusion because inhaling nature feels just so darn good.

1. Count each of your 12-18, slow, steady, smooth breaths and anchor yourself in present moment.

2. Aim for full exhalation, squeeze out every bit of breath, and feel yourself invite a self-inspired ease to your over-amped mind and body.

3. Make your very last exhale, your biggest and best. Sigh it all out, let it all go, smile, and carry on, resilient human that you are.

ANXIETY

I know what you're thinking, "Gosh this girl talks a lot about the breath." Why? Because it's that damn important.

- Firstly, when we breathe, we live... a major perk. And if we choose to be mindful of our breath in any given moment, life gets even better! Attending to our breath can ease symptoms of anxiety by compelling us to remain rock solid in the present moment, not stuck in the past, beating ourselves up, or consumed by worries of an unknown future, but rather, being right here, right now.

- Secondly, a single moment in time is far more manageable than many moments lumped together in one giant overwhelming clusterfuck of regret and fear. When we are in crisis, we lack perspective.

- Lastly, slowing down the breath and extending the exhalation can literally shift the physiology of anxiety, by inviting ease to a ramped up nervous system, turning down the volume on fight-flight-freeze-fawn, and turning up the volume on rest-digest-rejuvenate. We can shift ourselves from heart palpitations, sweats, body tremors, and monkey-mind into greater calmness in all layers of being. The breath: the gift that keeps on giving.

EXTENDED EXHALATION: THERAPEUTIC BREATH

- Invites ease and calms the nervous system

- Lowers anxiety levels

- Releases increased levels of carbon dioxide (toxins)

1. As you move through Three Part Breath, add an intentional count to both your inhale and exhale, whereby the exhale is just a little bit longer than your inhale.

2. Begin with an Inhale 4 Count, Exhale 6 Count.

3. If you have greater capacity, explore an Inhale 6 Count. Exhale 8 Count.

4. Do not force the exhale, as doing so could have the opposite affect and increase your stress response.

This do-it-anywhere breath will become one of your favorite go-to supports in your self-care toolkit.

Demo Video: Access "How to" in your RECLAIMED Library: https://bit.ly/accesslibrary

BEE BREATH / BRAHMARI

• Maintains healthy levels of CO_2 in the bloodstream

• Cultivates ease

• Calms anxiety

1. Make an "M" sound and buzz like a bee on your exhale.

2. Hands may rest comfortably on thighs, or you may seal off using the tragus, the little flaps of both ears, with your index fingers for a more inward experience.

3. Do for several minutes. The longer you do Bee Breath, the more relaxed you become.

4. Let your inhale resume naturally.

5. Don't force the exhale, as it may have the opposite effect, and increase your stress response.

6. When you have completed your rounds, allow yourself to sit for a few moments. Observe sensation and energy, receive the gifts of your breath practice.

Your on-the-spot remedy for anxiety.

ALTERNATE NOSTRIL BREATHING - NADI SHODHANA

- A mental state reset

- Restores the nervous system

- Calms anxiety

- Helps focus the mind

- Supports lung and respiratory function

- Balances the left and right hemispheres of the brain

- Eases stress

- Releases toxins

1. Close the eyes or keep open maintaining a soft, yogic gaze or drishti.

2. The right thumb will be used to seal the right nostril.

3. To settle in, inhale and exhale through the left nostril, slowly and steadily.

4. Now, inhale through the left nostril.

5. Seal the left nostril with your left index and middle finger, as you then open the right nostril to exhale.

6. Now, inhale through right nostril, and seal the right nostril with thumb as you then open the left nostril to exhale.

7. This is one cycle of alternate nostril breathing.

8. Repeat 5- 10 cycles. Soothe your soul with this one.

Demo Video: Access "How to" in your RECLAIMED Library: https://bit.ly/accesslibrary

UJJAYI: BREATH OF VICTORY

- A warming breath

- Invigorates and cultivates energy

- Infuses whole being with life force (prana)

- Restores and rejuvenates the nervous system

- Helpful if you are struggling with depression, low energy, lethargy, and lack of motivation

- Immunity booster

- Supports sleep

1. Moving through Three Part Breath, bring a slight constriction to the back of your throat. This will make the breath audible to you, perhaps, slightly audible to someone sitting next to you. We are not going for a Darth Vader breath here... ha! ha! I much prefer to think of it as the sound of the ocean in my ears.

2. If it is helpful, imagine holding up a mirror to your mouth and exhaling to fog up the glass.

3. As you practice, keep the breath mindful, slow, calm, fluid, and relaxing, not forcing or pushing.

4. Moving through 10–15 cycles at minimum, and up to 10–20 minutes daily for optimal benefit.

Need a swift kick in the rear-end? This breath has got your back and will get you moving!

KAPALABHATI

- Energy booster for body and mind

- Builds heat

- Releases toxins

- Improves digestion

- Invites clarity and focus of mind

- Tones diaphragm and core muscles

- Improves skin health and inspires a radiance

Kapalabhati is considered a more advanced breathing technique. So, begin with mastering your ujjayi. When this is feeling good, proceed with your exploration of Kapalabhati. In this pranayama, you will alternate short, forceful exhalations with longer, passive inhalations. Your powerful exhales will actively contract your lower belly, and then when the contraction is released the inhale naturally resumes with air drawn back into the lungs.

1. Begin by bringing awareness to your lower belly. It can be helpful to place or fist your hands on your belly.

2. Take a cleansing breath: easy inhale through the nose, easy exhale out through the mouth.

3. Now, inhale deeply to fill the belly, aim for ¾ full.

4. From here, much like a pump, repeat quick, short, forced exhales out through the nose (the passive inhales occur in between your exhales).

5. The movement is initiated by the diaphragm, and you want to feel the belly button draw into the spine with each explosive exhale. This is the contraction.

6. You can use your hands on the belly to support the "pumping" action.

7. Upon completion, pause and bring awareness to your breath and sensation.

8. Aim for 25- 30 cycles and build from here to 100 or more.

BREATH OF JOY

- Inspires joy

- Invigorates and cultivates energy

Breath of Joy is 3 quick sips of air in, with the coordinating arm movements, followed by one big, letting-go exhale, coordinated with arm movement and gentle squatting action. See the steps below.

1. Start from Standing Mountain Pose, Tadasana, with easy softness in your knees.

2. First sip of air: Arms sweep up and skyward in front of body.

3. Second sip of air: Arms sweep out and away from sides of body.

4. Third sip of air: Arms sweep up and skyward, again.

5. Then a big *letting-go* exhale, as arms sweep back down alongside body, and you simultaneously forward fold from the hip (bending knees, as needed to support tight upper back thighs, your hamstrings specifically), releasing the breath through the mouth as fully and as audibly as you wish.

6. This is one cycle. Aim for 5-10 cycles. When you complete the last round, stand up slowly, keeping your head up to prevent lightheadedness.

7. Return to Tadasana, with your eyes closed and gaze inward. Observe flow of breath, beat of heart... sensation. vibration in physical body.... energy... and mood.

8. Smile and gently open your eyes.

You may move through a second round of Breath of Joy at the same pace or, alternatively, get faster and faster, in both breath and movement, with each passing cycle.

May you inspire and find joy!

TO RECAP:

✓ You now know how to effect change to your breath for a desired outcome, to soothe the nervous system, invite ease, calm anxiety, decrease your pain level or, alternatively, empower energy and mobilize yourself.

✓ You are going to explore these at-your-fingertips pranayamas, to step into the driver's seat of your present-moment experience and give yourself what you need to shift gears.

✓ You are going to make a daily habit of breath awareness and connection. It is literally life force flowing through you, your most potent recovery tool.

✓ You understand that breath is life and life is breath. Yes, your breath is The Bomb!

✓ You are going to keep honing awareness, deepening connection, and taking mindful, purposeful action.

✓ YOU ARE LEARNING TO MAKE A DAILY HABIT OF INTENTIONAL BREATHING.

Now, that you're breathing easy, let us turn our attention to movement in the physical body. Firstly, we are going to talk about the principles of alignment that serve to inspire a practice of longevity.

Meet you next, in **Chapter 5: EmPOWERed Alignment**, building the framework for safe, feel-good movement.

"I have always known breath is important to health, I just did not realize how important. I also did not realize there are specific breathing techniques to help ease anxiety and depression. Bee Breath and Breath of Joy are now my go-tos, depending upon what I need, ie. to calm or to inspire energy."

- 1:1 Reclaimed Mastery Client

Darkness Is Afoot

You find your perch, you set your grip,
you insidiously weave yourself around every cell of my being

You hold me captive, blindfold, and bind me, there is no light,
I am immobilized

You lick your lips in maniacal delight, steadfast satisfaction,
as you make child's play of my vulnerability and shame

You taunt me, fastidiously devouring my heart, my mind, my
soul,
without care or conscience

You take what you want, leaving me vacant and bone-weary
exhausted

You are relentless in your pursuit; complete annihilation is
your end game

You are my most ferocious foe, my nemesis

It takes all I have to greet you, to rise up and meet you,
like the mighty warrior I know I must be

I fix my stance and bravely lift my sword,
inevitably it falls, it feels heavier this time,
and I feel so encumbered

I draw upon my full arsenal of resource

Years of self-reflection, self-work, digging even deeper this
time,
hoping beyond hope it is enough

I fight fiercely and ache for a new dawn

Days turn into nights, nights into days

This battle, our battle, is epic

In one last hurrah, I anchor myself in gratitude,
my battle cry is love, and I triumphantly raise my sword
to strike an almighty blow against you

You don't expect it, it hits with precision,
and you falter just long enough
for that first glimmer of light to break through

It is enough for me, and I strike again, and again, and again

Today, you are beaten, the victory is mine

I see you now, as you are

You are not real

You are not real

BUT I AM

From Julie's Journal & Journey

An extra special Mother's Day
May 13th, 2018

It's Mother's Day today, and I am feeling so very grateful. I woke in one of my very favorite places on earth with some of my favorite peeps; birds singing, the sound of surf upon the shore, blue skies, sunshine, and sweet, salty air. In marked contrast, less than six months ago I was recovering in hospital having attempted to take my own life. Those were truly my darkest days.

It was the end of November and I had been dreading my birthday all week. I did not feel deserving of being celebrated. In fact, I had spent the week convincing myself that my loved ones would be far better off without the complication of 'Julie' in their lives.

And if you are currently having this kind of inner dialogue with yourself, you need to hear me now, "You could not be further from the truth."

I woke up and moved heavily through my morning routine… make lunches… school drop-off… celebratory chai with family and friends at regular coffee haunt… then off to teach my yoga class. The thirty-minute drive to the studio was painful. Tears streamed, could barely breathe, called ahead to say I was enroute, but that I was a colossal mess. Taught my class, was celebrated in the traditional Birthday Yoga Chair, BIG SMILES, more chai and chat at Starbucks with one of my dearest friends. She asked if I was OK. I said, "Yes." Liar! And then I headed back home.

Now, I am seaside, listening to the sound of my son's laughter as he rides a wave to shore along with his best buddy. They live in different cities, go to different schools, but each year they reunite for this family holiday and, honestly, they do not skip a beat...they simply carry on from the year prior, one year older. It is a beautiful thing to see, to hear, and my heart feels full.

The drive home from the studio was a repeat performance... more tears... harder to breathe..., heart shattering in pieces. Got home, opened a thoughtful birthday present, and placed it on my desk with the gift receipt, along with the gift cards I had received. If I wasn't going to use them, I would leave them out for someone who could. Time to pick up my son from school. We drive home and I tell him how much I love him, how proud of him I am, that he is the very best thing I have ever done in my life... I tell him this often... but I found out later he heard something different in my voice that day. As we pull into driveway, I say to Ollie, "Tell Dad I am just going to pick up some cream for coffee."

Walking the beach now. It is a perfect day and people are walking, running, fishing. Full of joy. It's like coming home for me here and I can feel the healing power of this place in each breath I take, in each step I take. I feel lighter than I have in a long time. I feel alive.

I have tucked myself into the woods and lain down to die. I am incredibly tired. It is cold, a combination of rain and snow, and I am not dressed for winter. I am shivering but it does not deter me. I am ready to let go. Maybe it's a couple of hours later, not really sure, and I could not hear them calling me over the chattering of my teeth. Eventually I do hear, "We've got her and she's breathing. Julie, we understand you have been having a really tough go of things." I felt no relief in being found, more a resignation that today was not going to be the day. It was a police dog that found me, and the first responders involved in the search were beyond kind and compassionate. It made all the difference. I found out later, that it was due to swift action on my family's part that things moved so quickly… my husband, son, sister, mother, brother-in-law, niece, and stepfather all desperately coming together to battle for me with everything they had. A helicopter was going to be sent out, but weather conditions were not conducive. A police dog was the best option, but it was going to take forty-five minutes to get one on scene. It was enough time. And I was one lucky lady…even if I did not realize it at the time.

I am sitting on the deck, the view is perfection in every direction, and I am listening to the easy banter and laughter of dear family and friends, savoring every moment. Yes, the last few months have been excruciatingly hard, but this makes it all worth it.

I am now sitting with my husband, sister, and the intake crisis counselor, thawing out, bandaged, trying to make rhyme or reason of the day's events. I am ambivalent. I feel no relief in being alive…, if anything, disappointment. Yet, I recognize I should feel differently. This scares the shit out of me. Most pressing on my mind, "What kind of mother am I?" My crisis counselor says, "It is 'Unwell Julie' that got you here, not 'Healthy Julie'." It helps a little, but I continue to think, "What kind of mother am I?" My heart aches. I am wracked with guilt. I feel undeserving. Even in this moment, I feel I need to take responsibility for my decisions and actions. I do not wish to be let off the hook and I struggle to reconcile it all. Was this a remaining glimmer of 'Healthy Julie'?

In the days that follow it is my ambivalence that proves to be my greatest hurdle and I talk incessantly about it with my family, friends, nurses, and psychiatrist. I wish to feel the relief in my aliveness and gratitude that I get to look into my son's eyes, feel his arms around me, hear his laughter and bask in his love… I don't. I am neither here nor there. Dammit. What kind of mother am I? Doc' reminds me to be patient and kind with myself, "It will come, you are still 'Unwell Julie' fighting to free herself from that dark place and move into the light." As it turns out he was right… relief did come, but not without the really, really hard work.

Looking out at the sea with a keen awareness of the beauty that surrounds me, igniting my senses… sight… smell… sound… touch… taste. I am overwhelmed by this gift I have been given, a second chance. So very grateful!

Weeks and months pass, and I dig deeper than I ever have in my life… battling for myself… battling for Ollie…, battling my guilt… battling my depression and my anxiety…relentlessly and ferociously. And the healing and recovery? It is happening with each and every moment that passes. Is it freaking hard? Do I have setbacks? Hell, yes, but I am doing it, a daily effort and a daily celebration. What I have come to realize is… I AM a great mom, far from perfect, but still great! In moving through this experience with Ollie, I am leading by example, taking ownership and responsibility, part of which includes me diligently employing all my self-care tools… sleep, nutrition, yoga, exercise, meds, counselling… to prevent being sucked into 'The Vortex' of my depression. In so doing, I realize I am raising a soon-to-be 13-year-old young man who has a kindness and a compassion beyond his years. This is a young man who came home from school one day so excited to tell me, "Mom! Mom! You won't believe it! We were all talking in class today about this famous rapper who made a song whose title is the phone number people can call if they were at risk for suicide. Isn't this awesome Mom?! It has and it will help people that struggle like you struggled Mom!" When I tell you he did not stumble upon the word suicide, he did not. Of course, he was referring to Logic's 1-800-273-8255 featuring Alessia Cara and Khalid, and the highest-charting phone number in Billboard's Hot 100 History. This is the phone number for the National Suicide Prevention Lifeline in the United States. In being open and honest with Ollie, I can only hope he will learn to nurture both his physical and mental well-being, that he will seek support if he is in need, and be there for his friends, if and when the time comes, with love and non-judgement.

So, yes, today is an extra special Mother's Day. I am full of gratitude for this life, for my family, my friends, Ollie's teachers, Ollie's school, my yoga community, the community in which I live, my counselors, my nurses, my doctors, the first responders, my fellow patients, and for those of you who battle every day to meet your mental health struggles head on... you are all an inspiration. Fight the fight. You are worth it. We are worth it. Do not surrender. Do not give up. If you feel alone, trust me, you are not. You are loved and you are supported. Advocate for what you need and do not stop. Ever.

And now, it's time to hit the beach again, to breathe, to move, to play, to live. I am one lucky woman, indeed.

CHAPTER 5

EmPOWERed Alignment

*Movement is the unifying bond between
the mind and the body,
and sensations are the substance
of that bond.*
- Deane Juhan

Much of what we do has us working and playing in the front of our body... heads down... scrolling phones... staring at computer screens... commuting in cars... sitting at desks. Even the good stuff, walking, running, biking, you name it, has us hanging out in perpetual forward flexion... hinged forward from the hips, with chins projecting, compelling us away from our *optimal postural blueprint*. Yes, we have one! Not to mention, think about how this collapsed body shape compromises the flow of breath, the inhale limited to the upper levels of the chest, at best.

In yoga, the principles of alignment serve to return us home to our bodies and to set the foundation for safe, playful, exploratory movement. How we show up on our mats, physically, mentally-emotionally, energetically, and soulfully, will also determine the form our bodies take in any given moment. Body proportions and injury, with its compensatory movement patterns, will also impact the shape of our body in postures. What's the takeaway here?

Firstly, yoga should never hurt... EVER... we've heard this before, haven't we? Nudge edges mindfully... no forcing... no pushing... trust your intuition... trust yourself. You know your body best.

Secondly, can you keep... your breath calm... your body calm... your mind calm? Good rule of thumb: If one of these three things is compromised, give yourself permission to back off, or out of the posture, entirely. That's good yoga.

Lastly, stop 'should'ing yourself, as in, "I should look like this in my pose." You're not failing if your "shape" doesn't look exactly like the one on the cover of Yoga Journal. Instead, see yourself as the unique, beautiful, whole being that you are... your body... your practice... your expression.

We are now going to take some time to understand your optimal blueprint and explore various exercises to support you in returning to your most aligned self.

TADASANA - STANDING MOUNTAIN POSE – YOUR OPTIMAL BLUEPRINT

Breathe in, breathe out. Root evenly into all points of connection. Move from the middle, from center, literally and figuratively. Rise up from here, in your most grounded, supported, and strongest self. Breathe, be, believe, trust.

Building foundation from the ground up.

1. Come to stand with your feet hip-width apart (two fists width at backs of heels). Align the second toe with mid-ankle.

2. Lift and spread all ten toes. This is good for foot health. Mindfully root into big toe mound, inner heel, baby toe mound, outer heel, in this order. You will feel the arches of your feet lift. Maintain the energy, here, and bring toe pads down to meet the mat. You are rooting evenly into all four corners of the feet.

3. Hug your shins energetically toward the mid-line of the body, middle of kneecap remains aligned with the second toe. Nice soft knees, slight micro-bend, to keep your knees feeling supported and safe. Maintain this actioning throughout the exercise.

4. Your thigh bones (femur bones) will draw in back and apart. This will initiate a blossoming of your buttocks towards the back edge of your mat. Exaggerate this action. At the same time, you will draw the belly button in toward the spine to engage the lower, deeper transverse abdominals and soften the tailbone towards the earth, just the right amount. The goal here is to support you in settling into your *neutral pelvis*, but not so much that the tailbone begins to curl up and under. This will invite a spaciousness and support to your lower back. You will feel strong and supported, hanging in your *sweet spot*.

5. From here, lengthen through the spine and side body. Shoulders will draw away from the ears and away from the midline of the body, as your upper arm bones hug in toward mid-line of body. This will bring a broadening of your collar bone and a gentle lift of your heart skyward. Open your palms to the front of the room, thumbs drawing away from the mid-line, and imagine you are rooting actively into the pads of your fingers, base knuckles of fingers, and the heel of your hands, just as you have positioned your feet upon the mat. Our hands and feet serve as key points of connection, energy, and foundation for our movement exploration.

6. The base of the chin will remain parallel to the earth, as you draw the chin in towards the back of the head, to support neutral alignment of the cervical spine, your neck. Back of the neck lengthens and crown of the head floats skyward.

"Ta-da! Tadasana – Your Optimal Blueprint!" Breathe in. Breathe out. Notice how this feels. Some of it may feel uncomfortable, challenging, and that's OK. This is why yoga is a practice. It's a lot to think about, but eventually it becomes habitual, just as our misalignments have.

As the title indicates, "Tadasana in Every Asana." That is, in every posture you explore, Tadasana is the foundation for your movement exploration. The body is simply moving in a different orientation in space.

> **TRANSFORMATIONAL INSIGHT:** Whenever the body is misaligned the nervous system recognizes it as stress. Guess what this does to the nervous system? You got it, it keeps it in turbo mode and perpetuates our chronic pain experience.

So, with an open mind and an open heart, continue to practice and play with the foundational principles of alignment mindfully, and intentionally bring yourself back to your optimal blueprint relative to your physical structure and being.

This will keep you feeling... safe and spacious... breath flowing... joints integrated, supported, and stabilized.

This is how you begin to shift the story of pain and misalignment to one of freedom and alignment in all the layers of your being.

Demo Video: Access "How to Tadasana" in your RECLAIMED Library: https://bit.ly/accesslibrary

POSTURE FOUNDATION OPTIMIZER - P.F.O.

Intention: To support you in realigning the foundation of your posture from the ground up.

Exercise:

1. Have a yoga block in your hands.

2. Stand with your feet hip-width apart, second toe in front of mid-ankle. Lift and spread your toes, lift arches of feet, intentionally root into big toe mound, inner heel, baby toe mound, outer heel... in this order.

3. Align your spine in neutral.

4. Place hands on hips and bend your knees, bringing your mid-knee as wide as the mid-ankle. Squeeze the lower legs (shins) towards each other to engage and tone the inner leg muscles.

5. Place a block, narrow side and lengthwise between your thighs. Press your hands to the outer shins to help squeeze the lower legs towards the mid-line. Now, create resistance against the actions of the lower legs by squeezing the block and activating the upper thighs apart from each other. Your thigh bones draw in, back, and apart, and it will feel as if you are going to shoot the block straight out behind you.

6. From here, straighten the legs (not all the way straight) for a 5-count inhale and then bend the knees deeper (towards a squat) for a 5-count exhale.

IMPORTANT - Throughout the exercise...

• Maintain the resistance of the lower legs squeezing in, and the upper legs resisting apart

• Make sure the kneecaps stay aligned with mid-ankle - the block placement between thighs will help with this

• Keep toes and arches lifted

• Maintain neutral spine, do not flatten or round the back

*** If this exercise feels very intense and like a lot of work, you are doing it right! GO SLOW, with a 5-count inhale and a 5-count exhale to maximize results.

Demo Video: Access "How to" in your RECLAIMED Library: https://bit.ly/accesslibrary

"This (P.F.0.) is definitely challenging, but I find it gets easier and easier, as my body returns to and embraces its optimal way of being. I feel stronger and more aligned, not just physically, but mentally, too."
- Reclaimed Mastery Client

COSMIC HEAD REST

Intention: Reduce forward carriage of head and chin and support neutral re-alignment of the cervical spine (neck).

Note: Forward head carriage reduces lung capacity by 30%. It creates lack of cervical lordosis, tight pectorals and trapezius muscles, and inhibition of the rhomboids.

Exercise:

1. This posture may be explored lying down, seated, or standing.

2. Interlace your fingers and place them behind your head at the base of the skull (little bump called the occipital bone).

3. Align spine and neck in neutral.

4. Pull your shoulders down, back, and away from the midline, broadening collar bone and lifting heart skyward - think about wrapping your shoulder blades around the back of your heart, firmly.

5. Press your head back while resisting with the hands, as you simultaneously draw (gently) upward with the hands at the base of the skull, lengthening the neck and creating space between the vertebrae.

6. Breathe here for several smooth breaths.

Worth Repeating: Whenever the body is misaligned, the nervous system recognizes it as stress.

"My neck has always been a hot spot for me in terms of pain. Cosmic Head Rest has become a daily practice for me and resulted in lesser to no pain at all. 5 stars!"
- Reclaimed Mastery Client

SPINAL BALANCING - TABLE POSE VARIATION

Intention: Strengthen and stabilize the spine, core activation.

Exercise:

1. Come to hands and knees, Table Pose... shoulders and wrists stack... knees and hips stack... toes curled under... feet square to back edge of mat.

2. Gaze toward front edge of mat to maintain neutral cervical spine... back of neck lengthening... crown of head extending.

3. Step back with the right leg and root intentionally into big toe and baby toe mound. Invigorate thigh. Inhale and lift right leg toward hip height... toes pointed toward mat... lift left arm toward shoulder height... thumb skyward... palm toward mid-line. Hold for 3-5 breaths. On the fifth exhale, lower the right leg and come back to table pose.

4. Step back with the left leg and root intentionally into big toe and baby toe mound. Invigorate thigh. Inhale and lift left leg toward hip height... toes pointed toward mat... lift right arm toward shoulder height... thumb skyward... palm toward mid-line. Hold for 3-5 breaths. On the fifth exhale, lower the left leg and come back to table pose. Roll your wrists and repeat if you wish.

Practice Tip: If lifting the leg is challenging for you right now, simply remain rooted in the big toe mound, baby toe mound of the extended leg and lift the corresponding arm, accordingly. Work in the range of motion that feels just right for you.

IMPORTANT: Throughout the exercise:

- Maintain neutral spine position along the full length of your spine

- Keep your hips as square as possible with your mat

- Lengthen through spine and side body, tone lowest belly

- Muscle energy draws in towards the midline to support stability

Have fun with this one. Imagine that you are trying to balance teacups on your back.

BOOST YOUR BOUNDARIES

Setting healthy boundaries is an act of love.
A form of respect for self, for others.

Definition: Boundaries

"Boundaries define what is me and what is not me. A boundary shows me where I end and someone else begins."[7]

Just as Tadasana (Standing Mountain Pose) supports empowered alignment in our movement practice, so does the effective use of boundaries support our optimal blueprint relative to our relationship with both self and others.

Key Boundary Types

For our purposes, we are going to highlight four key boundary types and what needs or aspects of life and relationship they address.

Physical

- Eating

- Hydrating

- Exercising

---

7   Henry Cloud and John Townsend, *Boundaries: When to Say Yes, How to Say No to Take Control of Your Life* (New York: Zondervan, 1992), 13-14

- Resting

- Personal space

- Touch

Sample Boundary Statements:

1. "I will not work through my lunch, but rather set 30 minutes aside to nourish myself with good food and hydration."

2. "I know you would like me to meet you for dinner, but I am committed to the gym tonight."

3. "We talked about meeting early for coffee Saturday morning, but it's been a tough week and I am going to sleep in and ease into my day."

4. "I am not a hugger, but good for an enthusiastic fist pump!"

Emotional

- Feelings

- Emotional energy

- Being selective with whom we share our feelings and emotional energy

- Validating our own and others' feelings

- Respecting capacity to receive emotional energy, both self and others

- Recognizing we cannot be all things to all people all of the time

Sample Boundary Statements:

1. "Please don't speak to me in that tone. It hurts my feelings and leaves me feeling disrespected."

2. "I know you are struggling deeply, and I remain here for you. However, I feel my capacity to support you, effectively, exceeds my expertise. I would like to recommend you seek out a psychotherapist."

Time

- Time is precious and must be safeguarded

- Intentional use of time at work, home, and play

- Clarity around priorities and not over committing

- Choosing not to "give away" our time to people-please, to meet others' needs and expectations at our own expense

Sample Boundary Statements:

1. "Our meeting is always scheduled for 10 a.m. and you are consistently late. I would ask that you respect my time and arrive on time moving forward."

2. "I would like to ask you to wake up early enough, so you have time to walk to school. When you are running late and need a ride, I end up shortening or missing my yoga practice. Yoga is one of the ways Mom sets her day up for success and I would like your support."

Intellectual

- Honoring our own and others' thoughts, ideas, and inquisitiveness

- Feeling seen, heard, acknowledged, and respected

- Retaining an open mind and heart for constructive conversation versus dismissive, demeaning, and judgmental comments

- Picking the right time for dialogue

Sample Boundary Statements:

1. "When you interrupt and speak over me, I feel what I am saying is not important and what you have to say is more important. May I ask that you give me the opportunity to finish my sentence?"

2. "I don't appreciate when you e-mail me racist jokes and comments. Please refrain from doing so. If it continues, I will have to block you."

3. "I appreciate you have your opinion on what I should do, however, this is how I feel about the situation, and I would ask that you respect my choice. I will extend the same courtesy to you."

THE DOWNSIDE OF NO BOUNDARIES

- Overcommitting yourself

- People-pleasing at your own expense

- Never feeling like you are enough or can do enough

- Acting from obligation vs choice

- Stress

- Exhaustion

- Impaired physical and/or mental-emotional health

- Resentment

- Feeling disempowered, used, and abused

- Feeling taken for granted, under-appreciated

- Encouraging codependent relationships

THE UPSIDE OF BOOSTED BOUNDARIES

- Awareness that your time and energy are respected

- Ability to show up for others with intention

- Confidence speaking your truth, asking for what you need

- Authenticity

- Self-awareness and connection

- Clarity and calm

- Feeling seen, heard, acknowledged, and valued

- Feeling respected by self and others

- Enjoying mutually rewarding, fulfilling relationships

- Capacity to let go relationships where your boundaries are repeatedly violated, or where there is a significant difference in your core values

EXERCISE: BOOST YOUR BOUNDARIES

1. Identify the key relationships in your life... personally... professionally... with community... with nature... as applicable. Write them down.

2. In each of these relationships, what boundaries, if any, do you consciously have in place to support mutually healthy, respectful, rewarding engagement? Write these down as Current Boundaries.

3. Are these current boundaries doing the job? Are they creating flow and fulfilling interactions? Notice where feelings of resistance exist (awareness). Mark each boundary with a '✓' for YES (serving me) and an 'X' for NO (not serving me). For those marked X, take a moment to reflect...

    -   Is it lack of follow through?

    -   Does the boundary itself lack clarity and efficacy?

    -   Is there opportunity to create an improved or new boundary?

4. Take time to brainstorm... to get crystal clear... to find just the right wording.

    -   Write these boundaries down

    -   Sit with them

    -   Try them on

    -   Practice articulating... implementing... upholding them... in your relationships

- Get comfortable and confident asking for what you need and with saying NO.

- This may be in the form of direct conversation, a letter, or even leading by example. Sometimes we need to show people what we need.

5. Keep an open mind and heart.

6. Your boundaries may require tweaking as you put them into daily action.

"The only people who get upset when you set boundaries are the ones who benefited from you having none." – Unknown

TO RECAP:

✓ You have your very own optimal blueprint. Over the course of time, you are pulled away from this *sweet spot* in your physical body, due to lack of awareness, injury, and/or compensatory movement patterns.

✓ You now understand that whenever the body is misaligned the nervous system recognizes it as stress, and this perpetuates the chronic pain experience.

✓ You now have the tools to begin to kindly invite your body back to its blissful baseline.

✓ You are going to keep honing awareness, deepening connection, and taking mindful, purposeful action.

- ✓ You have the means to create clarity around your personal boundaries, to practice asking for what you need and saying, "NO." When necessary, you can choose to let go of relationships where your boundaries are consistently violated. You have the means to extend to others what you seek for yourself relative to their boundaries
- ✓ YOU ARE LEARNING TO MAKE A DAILY HABIT OF BEING AND BREATHING IN YOUR OPTIMAL BLUEPRINT, PHYSICALLY, MENTALLY-EMOTIONALLY, ENERGETICALLY, AND SOULFULLY.

We now have a good grasp on the principles of alignment, and how they support the framework from which we may explore movement safely, constructively, freely, and playfully.

We also have a deeper understanding of the necessity of boundaries to support our optimal blueprint relative to our relationship with both ourselves and others.

Next, we turn our attention to Kind Movement practices and why less is more when it comes to sustainable healing and recovery. It just keeps getting better and better. Can you feel it?

"Julie encouraged me to play in the poses, and to start to listen to what tiny adjustments made my body sing. Through miniscule movements, I started to feel at home in my body."

- Reclaimed Mastery Client

"Hey! It felt so very good. I felt new after and was able to exchange in a nicer way with everyone. And my body felt awesome – I was so aware of it!"

- Reclaimed Mastery Client

From Julie's Journal & Journey

Go get it, whatever it takes
June 4th, 2018

How do we ease anxiety and rise out of depression? We do this by choosing to do whatever it takes to inspire our own healing and recovery. Maybe we need to breathe differently... delve deeper into mindfulness... check out meditation... or move differently, e.g., yoga, walk, run, bike, hike, qigong, take up Kung Fu, salsa dance, play in the garden, paddleboard... whatever floats our boat. Eat differently (better, more, less)... nourish and hydrate... read more... sleep longer... sleep less... talk more and to the right people... talk less and listen more, again, to the right people... maybe we find ourselves a counsellor, and if it's not a good fit, we don't stop the search until we find the one that is... maybe we check out group counseling and we say "yay" or "nay"... maybe we consider medications that help us take the edge off, give ourselves the space to cope and to do what must be done to impel movement forward... maybe we are already on meds and they are doing the job or perhaps they are exacerbating current symptoms and/or creating new ones. Again, we have a choice. We advocate for ourselves, we go to our psychiatrist and say, "Hey, I don't feel right."

Case in point: I started on a new medication, during my hospital stay, to help bring balance to my mood and ease my anxiety. Within a few weeks I was 'seeing red' literally. Rage has never, ever been a part of my mental health symptomology, nor has it been part of my day-to-day modus operandi. Let me tell you, I was one short fuse... instantaneous rage. I did not recognize myself and knew something wasn't right. This prompted me to speak with my Doc' and, under his guidance, I weaned myself off. Eventually, and with much relief, I might add, the green hue of my skin began to fade, and I was able to kick my inner 'Hulkster' to the curb!

All of the above, some of the above, none of the above may be helpful in navigating our journey with mental health, and what ends up working may completely surprise us. The fact remains that healing and recovery lie within our very own hands. If we knew that a resource, a tool, a lifestyle change could ease discomfort, sadness, and pain, and move us towards contentment, joy, and freedom, would it not be worth giving it a try? And it goes without saying, some of the things we choose to explore in our self-care strategy may not always become part of the solution, but many absolutely will, with symptoms diminishing, maybe even disappearing. How freaking awesome will that feel?

Your well-being, your mental health. Whatever it takes, however long it takes. Leave no stone un-turned. You are worth it.

CHAPTER 6

Kind Movement

Move your body kindly, compassionately, patiently, In every direction. Whenever you can, wherever you can, however you can.

Starting with the obvious, I love the movement in yoga. It is what initially compelled me to the practice. Like many North Americans, I was seeking another hardcore work-out to add to my 'more is more' philosophy. Instead, I got schooled, big time, in the value of less is more. What happens when we choose to settle mindfully into what I refer to as kind, moderate movement? We cultivate greater awareness. We attend more effectively to sensation in our bodies. We connect more deeply to our experience, and it is through this connection that we inspire invaluable, purposeful action. What we gift ourselves in return is less pain and discomfort. We invite ease, space, expansion, and equanimity. And the breath, our life force energy, flows more freely, bringing nourishment and union to all the layers of our being. This is the magic of yoga. And I can tell you this, without a doubt, I am in the best shape of my life, as compared to, way back when, when I was *enthusiastically* pumping iron and running myself into the ground, plagued by subsequent overuse ailments and injury.

There are many forms of yoga and teaching styles out there, from which you can choose. Begin by finding what feels just right for you in this moment. Remember, it is always your practice. Trust your intuition. Listen to your body. Be kind. And never force or push. YOGA SHOULD NEVER HURT. Read this again, please.

And if you are currently limited in your capacity to move, due to acute injury or chronic pain, begin by visualizing yourself moving in all the ways you wish to move. This reflects powerful intention and is scientifically proven to have a similar effect upon your healing to the movement itself.

WHAT IS ASANA ANYWAY?

Making shapes that make sense, and feel good, in that moment. It's that simple.

I often refer to the *sweet spot* when I teach yoga, and if your mind has segued, please come back to me now--ha! ha! The *sweet spot*, yogically speaking, is meeting that edge of your posture/asana, where you can continue to keep your breath calm, body calm, and mind calm. If any of these three things is compromised in the exploration of a posture/asana, it is likely you may be pushing too hard... short term pain for long term pain, perhaps even injury. The key here is to back off just enough to return to a state of ease, giving time and space for breath to flow and musculature and connective tissue to safely let go. Trust me when I tell you, you will begin to experience great growth in all aspects of your yoga practice, physically, mentally, emotionally, and soulfully.

Take this theory off your mat and you also have a great metaphor for life. Think twice about kicking the door down to manage challenges, discomforts, resistance, and tensions. Doing this may result in some short-term relief, but not necessarily the outcome you truly desire or deserve. Instead try backing off, breathing and being in the *sweet spot*, kindly, compassionately, patiently.

All right, let's have a look at some of my tried-and-trues when it comes to supporting my clients with kind movement.

LEGS UP THE WALL

If you do one yoga asana, make it this one.

The most parasympathetic pose of them all... pure magic!

Legs Up the Wall is a restorative inversion that packs a powerful, peaceful punch.

Key benefits include:

- Calms anxiety

- Relieves symptoms of mild depression and insomnia

- Relieves mild backache

- Restores tired, cramped legs and feet

- Passively stretches the back of the neck, front torso, and back of the legs

- Regulates blood flow

- Lowers blood pressure

- Improves digestion

- Provides migraine and headache relief

Any amount of time spent in Legs Up the Wall is golden. However, from a restorative standpoint, settling in for 15-30 minutes is optimal. Why? It is believed, once we move beyond the 15-minute mark, the volume is turned down on the sympathetic nervous system... fight-flight-freeze-fawn and the volume is turned up on the parasympathetic nervous system... *rest-digest-rejuvenate*. This shift is a welcome reprieve for our constantly amped up nervous systems and invites all the amazing benefits above, and more! The longer we hang out here, the greater the restoration.

Practice tips:

1. To support your lower back, place a folded blanket beneath your sacral area, the flat space just beneath the natural curvature of your low back.

2. Bring your buttocks to meet the wall and roll to your back body, as you extend your legs up the wall.

3. If your upper back of thighs (hamstrings) is tight, move your buttocks away from the wall, just enough to invite more space and ease to your back body.

4. If your feet fall asleep you may gently roll your ankles, wiggle your toes; or bend through your knees and bring your feet to rest upon the wall.

5. Place a folded blanket across your pelvis, such that its weight invites a deeper sense of grounding and connection... and it just feels so-o-o darn good.

6. When exploring restoratively to the best of your ability, aim to settle into stillness in both mind and body, let gravity do the work.

This is definitely a must-have in your self-care arsenal. Breathe, be, and receive its wealth of gifts!

FORWARD FOLDS & BACKBENDS – RULE OF THUMB

1. Forward folds soothe the nervous system and calm anxiety.

2. Standing forward folds versus seated forward folds tend to be the better option if you are struggling with back and/or hip pain.

3. Backbends are energy inspiring. They build heat and help manage depression and lethargy.

Choose the movement that serves you best in any given moment and give yourself what you need.

KAYA KRIYA

This action, although it may appear simple on the surface, is a powerful practice for releasing mental and physical tension, as well as providing relief from physical traumas and body pain. It is also good for those who suffer from anxiety. And is an ideal technique in yoga for insomnia.

Watch the video for the *ins and outs* on this one. In the beginning, it will feel a little like tapping your head and rubbing your belly at the same time - ha! ha! Be playful and patient with yourself. Don't get too hung up on perfect execution. Just keep breathing, being, and moving.

I utilize this yoga tool all the time. I even do it lying in bed!

The simultaneous, gentle movement at the joints (ankles, hips, shoulders, neck), combined with the breath, makes this a very soothing and powerful Present Moment Practice aka 'PMP' for short!

▶ **Demo Video:** Access "How to" in your RECLAIMED Library: https://bit.ly/accesslibrary

WALK DON'T RUN

This is one of my key healing and recovery hacks. Let's talk walking, preferably in the fresh air, not only as a highly effective form of low impact, less-is-more physical exercise, but as a powerful moving meditation that can invigorate your mental well-being and profoundly inspire your creativity.-

Along with yoga, walking has been one of the most powerful tools I have drawn upon to support my personal healing journey and mental health recovery. Kilometer after kilometer of... wild-wandering... body-grooving... heart-pumping... fresh air-breathing... vitamin D-receiving... mind-reflecting... soul-igniting... life-liberating exploration! If I tally it all up, I am quite sure I have walked coast-to-coast at least twice, maybe even three times... ha! ha!

So, if walking is not currently part of your self-care toolkit, I gently encourage you to grab your sneakers... maybe a buddy... maybe some great tunes... better yet, savor the sweet sounds of nature... and put one fabulous foot in front of the other. You may find yourself joyfully striding and pleasantly surprised by where your path leads you. Happy trails!

If you are just getting started, go slow. Maybe it's a slow stroll around the block, and from here building up your time, consistency, and pace. When I work with my clients, I recommend aiming for 3-5 times per week, 15-60 minutes in duration, depending upon time available. The key is to make it doable. You may even pepper your day with multiple short, sweet little walks! Remember your *islands of calm*?

And now, the best part. I am delighted to offer you two kind movement practices to explore at your own pace. With love from me to you!

INTUITIVE FLOW PRACTICE

The intention behind this breath and movement exploration is just that: to exercise your muscle of intuition, connecting to it deeply, trusting it, empowering mindful, purposeful action, and impelling yourself towards your optimal state of being - meeting the ebb and flow of life with grace, equanimity, and capacity.

1. Always work at your own pace, within your pain-free range of motion.

2. Keep your... breath calm... body calm... mind calm. as you move through your practice. If any one of these three things is compromised, you are likely pushing too hard. Kindly acknowledge this... breathe in... breath out... and mindfully release the posture. Settle into a place and space that feels just right for you, maybe a child's pose, savasana, easy-cross legged pose.

3. Do part or all this practice, depending upon how you feel. Remember, there is no place you have to be in your practice. It is your practice, always.

4. Practice *Tadasana in every asana*, your foundational principles of alignment to draw yourself back to your optimal blueprint, physically, mentally, emotionally, energetically, and making it habitual and natural.

5. Explore kindly, compassionately, patiently, lovingly, and playfully.

I am with you in each breath and movement, sharing energy and intention.

Demo Video: Access "Intuitive Flow Practice" in your RECLAIMED Library: https://bit.ly/accesslibrary

BLISS THIS YIN & RESTORATIVE PRACTICE

Now, we are going to slow things right down. In its entirety, this offering is on the longer, more luxurious side of time. It's jam-packed with goodness. If you have the time to gift yourself its full length, absolutely do so. All the layers of your being will thank you. It is 'workshoppy' in nature, so you are more than welcome to practice parts of it depending upon what you feel you need.

Yin Component

The intention behind Yin is longer-hold postures focused on the lower body and spine whilst working, more specifically, in the connective tissue of the body. Postures are held for 3-5 minutes generally, and the edges of movement are nudged over time to support a slow release of the connective tissue... inspiring spaciousness and a deep and present moment exploration of breath, body, mind, energy, and soul.

Restorative Component

The intention behind *Restorative* is to settle into stillness... as much as the body can settle into stillness for an extended time... whilst supporting the body fully, utilizing yoga blocks, bolsters, and blankets. In essence, we let gravity do the work for us, as we lie back and receive the gifts. It is believed that it is at the 15-minute mark of 'working' restoratively that the volume is *turned down* on the sympathetic nervous system (*flight, fight, freeze, fawn*) and 'turned up' on the parasympathetic nervous system (rest, digest, restore, rejuvenate). This shift is a welcome reprieve for our amped up nervous systems. So, the longer we hang out the greater the restoration. For example, if we practice a restorative pose for 20 minutes, we have spent five magical minutes settling into the parasympathetic experience. Healing happens here. Single restorative yoga postures may be explored for up to 60 minutes or postures may be explored collectively in a 60-90 minutes class format.

You Will Need: A bolster, 2 blocks (4, if you have them, or two cushions can work), a blanket or two or three.

Practice Tips:

1. Working yin-like and restoratively tends to be a *cooling practice*. Body temperature drops as time passes, so wear layers and have those extra blankets handy. Tuck in, and always work at your pace, within your pain-free range of motion.

2. For many, the most challenging or uncomfortable aspect of yin and restorative practice is the capacity to remain present when you hold postures for an extended period. If you find your mind wandering, such as making your grocery list. Trust me, it happens. Simply notice without judgement and kindly draw yourself back to breath and sensation in your physical body. Being present is a practice as well.

3. Keep your breath calm... your body calm... your mind calm... as you move through your practice. If any one of these three things is compromised, you are likely pushing too hard. Kindly acknowledge this... breathe in... breath out... and mindfully release the posture. Settle into a place and space that feels just right for you, maybe a child's pose, savasana, easy-cross legged pose, and rejoin the practice as you feel ready.

4. Do part, or all, of this practice, depending upon how you feel. Remember, there is no place you need to be in your practice. It is your practice, always.

5. The intention here is ease, softness, and spaciousness. Where appropriate, continue to practice your foundational principles of alignment, to draw yourself back to your optimal blueprint, physically, mentally-emotionally, energetically, and making it habitual and natural. We are laying new neural pathways here, and that takes repetition and practice.

6. Explore kindly, compassionately, patiently, lovingly, and playfully.

I am with you in each breath and movement, sharing energy and intention.

> **Demo Video:** Access "Bliss This Yin & Restorative Practice" in your RECLAIMED Library: https://bit.ly/accesslibrary

TO RECAP:

✓ You understand that less is almost always more when it comes to healing.

✓ You know that asana in yoga is simply about making shapes that make sense, and feel good, in that moment of time.

✓ You know that we can explore certain movements to invite a desired outcome in body and mind. For example, forward folds can ease anxiety and chronic pain states. Backbends can mitigate depression and increase energy.

✓ You now know the key... kind movement practices... what I use most often to effectively support my clients in their recovery journey.

✓ You are going to keep honing awareness, deepening connection, and taking mindful, purposeful action.

✓ YOU ARE LEARNING TO MAKE A DAILY HABIT OF LESS IS MORE.

We are in the process of creating multiple doorways through which we may move to support pain-free living and life reclamation. Little teaser... did you know that, like our *Optimal Physical Blueprint*, we have an *Energetic Blueprint*? Say what? Introducing **Chapter 7: Rock Your Chakras**... the next doorway. Let's crack this one open!

"There is a certain energy in women who own their lives, and it attracts attention from all. Julie is one of these women. I remember shopping in her clothing store and wishing we were friends and hearing her laugh at a local cafe and I would end up smiling myself. I swear I am not a stalker, we were just peripherally in the same group, in a small town, and Julie radiated energy.

It wasn't until years later when I had my first yoga class with Julie. I went in prepared to rock it. I was a 20-something woman with a lot of flexibility and could throw my body into just about any shape required. I was shocked to learn that yoga wasn't simply a stretch class. I had been doing it wrong all along. Julie challenged me to pull back from extreme range of motion in my hips and shoulders. Alternatively, she suggested I seek balance and stabilization using my muscles to hold a more neutral position. I'd had no idea that I could feel this much work happening in my body whilst doing so little. I continued with Julie's yoga classes as my fiancé was recovering from a significant injury, and yoga was the only thing I was doing for myself. I felt a little bit more like myself with each long, slow class.

One morning we targeted hip flexors, and I lost it. It is said the psoas muscle holds trauma and emotions, and as I loosened my muscles and settled into class, I wept for the year I was expecting to have... for our future marriage... for myself. I wept and wept. Julie first encouraged me to rest on my mat, and then when I was still sobbing after class, she sat with me and held me and handed me Kleenex after Kleenex. I couldn't tell you how long I cried for, I believe it was an hour or so past when class ended, and to this day I have never again been the recipient of such tenderness. When I think back on that day, I think of it as the day I felt cleansed, and the day I experienced true female empowerment and strength. Julie let me be fully myself, fully in my grief, and never made me feel as if this was shameful.

It wasn't until years later, writing this, I can appreciate the restraint and true kindness she showed by not ushering me through my feelings or offering suggestions. She showed up in the truest way and gifted me space. Life happened and while I am sure I returned to yoga for a bit after that day, our life took us elsewhere. It wasn't until nearly 6 years later that I realized that *that morning was the turning point in my life*. At the time it was a refreshing release, but not more. Six years later, having committed to some in-depth counseling and working through my portion of *family of origin* stuff, my counselor suggested I take up yoga to reconnect with my body. Quite honestly, I was not into the suggestion. My body had somehow become less and less my own throughout my life, harmed initially by sexual assault and *purity culture*, followed by feeling victimized by the medical system during pregnancy and giving birth, and the loss of self that often evolves with a little one at home. I was afraid of what I would learn if I noticed my body and I was confident I had no time. I was not going to do yoga.

Fortunately, I am driven by a need to be an A+ student, and as much as I refused to do yoga, I was obviously going to find a way to do yoga. As I sat with this suggestion, and journaled through my objections, I was left thinking of that day, way back when, where I sobbed on a yoga mat and Julie sat with me. If I was going to get in touch with my body, I was going to need someone as brave as Julie to go with me.

After a few frantic email exchanges and a fabulous re-meet and greet, I was signed up for the RECLAIMED program. I originally discounted this program at first glance because I didn't think I was dealing with pain or chronic illness. It was just my anxiety, and depression, and exhaustion, and an eye condition that might be an immune disease, and some random skin reactions to stress, and a short temper. Basically, I figured I was normal. What I knew I wanted was more of how Julie lives, and this seemed like a great way to get there.

The coaching side of the program is outstanding. With a few small exercises each day Julie had me noticing my body and my breath. We worked through gratitude, and my values and purpose in the world. We talked through the things that were ramping up my stress in everyday life and brainstormed ways to respond differently. We laughed a lot, I cried more than I expected, and the time always flew by.

For me, the magic was found on the mat. My body felt dangerous to me. Noticing it came with shame for all the days I had prioritized other people over myself. Moving through common poses like downward dog and cat cow, left me feeling vulnerable and afraid. I didn't feel strong, I felt like I was having a panic attack.

Again, as she had years earlier, Julie sat with me and let me cry. When I was ready, she let me talk and she took every word to heart. She came back to our next movement session with ideas of how to alter poses such that I could feel safe doing them. We moved slowly and we breathed deeply. Julie encouraged me to play in the poses, and to start to listen to what angles or tiny adjustments made my body sing. Through miniscule movements I started to feel at home in my body. We worked through alignment and Julie continued to find ways to tailor my poses so that they wouldn't spike my fight, flight, response.

There's no way to explain it, but things shifted for me. As I walked and practiced yoga, and played with my daughter, I felt a bit more and more myself. I looked in the mirror a bit longer and noticed my own face. It was such small shifts on any one day that I don't know if I noticed it happening. And then one day I showed up to yoga in a crop top. I went to the beach with my family and didn't feel the need to apologize or cover up. My body is mine and has carried me through 30-something years and a beautiful life. It's more my own now than it has ever been, and I love my body deeply. As she had years earlier, Julie helped me reframe success. I no longer need to throw my body in absurd shapes with an extreme range of motion to feel like I am working out. I get joy from feeling strength, as I focus on alignment and using my muscles to hold stable positions. It's a bit of a microcosm of how I have been reframing success throughout this whole program. I just want to have the capacity to feel steady, no matter which position I am in. I'm tired of the highs and lows, and I'm grateful for learning to use my mind and breath and body to build space for my own joy."

- Reclaimed Mastery Client

From Julie's Journal
& Journey

Landing and standing
on my own two feet
June 14th, 2018

Be sure you put your feet in the right place,
then stand firm.
– Abraham Lincoln

Over the course of the last few years, somewhere along the line, I lost my capacity to stand on my own two feet. I arrived at a place where I no longer believed I was 'enough' or honestly, strong enough to do so. I suddenly looked around one day and realized I was knee-deep in codependent relationships; where, in some cases, my lesser effective ways of being in the world were being enabled.

Part of my healing over the past few months has had me holding up the proverbial mirror and being brutally honest with myself... tough stuff... you bet. In seeking to empower myself, mentally, emotionally, soulfully, and financially within these relationships, I have been both humbled and liberated. In some instances, a change or a letting go of certain relationships has been necessary to create the space for exploration and growth.

The reward? In moving through this journey, I feel myself cultivating far healthier relationships, and a greater sense of autonomy, authenticity, balance, and freedom. Additionally, I am finding my voice and learning to articulate my needs... kindly, clearly, confidently, and consistently. As with anything else, it takes practice to shift behaviors and to support positive, permanent life change. One thing I know for sure, the landing and standing on my own two feet is beginning to feel pretty damn awesome!

Thus, my wish for you is simply that you choose to hold yourself, always, in the highest esteem and that you continue to fall madly, deeply, and unwaveringly in love with yourself. With this delightful treasure tucked securely in your self-care arsenal, then balanced, mutually rewarding and inspiring relationships become the icing, maybe even the 'cherry on top', of the cake of your sweet life.

CHAPTER 7

Rock Your Chakras!

It is up to us, how we explore the great wonders in our body, its life force, and subtle centers we call "CHAKRAS". We can either deny that they exist or learn to understand, work, and awaken them in order to live a more fulfilling life on planet Earth.
- Raju Ramanathan

DEFINITIONS:

The Chakra System

Your Energetic Blueprint... yes, you have one! It is also known as the Subtle Body. The word chakra means wheel, referencing wheels of energy throughout the body[8]. Harish Johari, author of the book *Chakras: Energy Centers of Transformation*, describes chakras as centers for transforming mental-emotional energy into spiritual energy.[9] My teacher, Kristine Kaoverii Weber, refers to the chakras (pronounced like you are saying chocolate chip cookies or, in this case, chakra-chip cookies) as the holographic

---

8 Parita Shah, "A Primer of the Chakra System", Chopra, https://chopra.com/articles/what-is-a-chakra

9 Harish Johari, *Chakras: Energy Centers of Transformation* (Rochester, Vermont: Destiny Books, September 1, 2000)

energetic blueprint of the physical body, as well as mind and spirit, where consciousness plugs into the body.[10]

Mudra

A symbolic hand gesture to intentionally channel the flow of energy, prana (life force).

Settling into a comfortable position, be it standing, seated, or lying down... eyes closed or eyes open with a soft gaze referred to as *drishti*... and a gentle awareness of breath, as you initiate the mudra. Keep in mind, many different mudras may be utilized for balancing a particular chakra, depending upon the intention behind it.

Affirmation

A means to constructively reprogram mindset using intentional, repetitive, self-empowering statements to foster belief in the actualization of a desired state of being and/or outcome.

In North America, we speak to the presence of seven chakras reflected energetically in the body. There are actually 114. For our purposes we will focus our exploration on the Seven Chakras:

1. Root Chakra
2. Sacral Chakra
3. Solar Plexus Chakra

---

10 Kristine Kaoverii Weber, "Yoga Cosmology, Psychology & The Chakras", Satva Health LLC, 2012

4. Heart Chakra
5. Throat Chakra
6. Third Eye Chakra
7. Crown Chakra

Each chakra has a location in the body, an element, and a color with which it is associated. We can also utilize specific breathing techniques, kind movement, mudra, and affirmation, to support a restoration of balance. Imbalance may be reflected by an overactive or underactive chakra. It is also important to note that the chakras do not exist in a vacuum, but rather are inextricably linked. A vulnerability in one chakra will affect the other six chakras. This is why it is so important to address the whole being when we are moving through healing and recovery.

In this introduction to the chakra system, you will gain clarity as to how to balance your chakras for optimal, whole health, and vitality.

OK. Here we go, the chakras in a nutshell!

ROOT CHAKRA

Located at the base of the spine (tailbone) this chakra reflects our sense of feeling grounded, safe, secure, and stable. It's about meeting our basic needs of life and survival. Remember, for healing to happen, we must first feel safe. If we are struggling with an imbalance here, we may feel unstable, untethered, and fearful. Now, take a moment to think about the impact upon the nervous system. Yep, you got it, it exacerbates our fight-flight-freeze-fawn response. So, how else might this show up in our physical and mental-emotional beings? It manifests...

In the body as:

- Tailbone issues
- Sciatica
- Lower body discomfort; legs, knees, feet
- Osteoarthritis
- Compromised immune system
- Constipation

In the mind and heart as:

- Eating disorders
- Anxiety
- Panic
- Fear
- Insecurity
- A feeling that survival is at risk

Element	: Earth
Color	: Red
Pranayama	: Alternate Nostril Breathing
Movement Focus	: Grounding poses and standing postures, such as easy pose, child's pose, standing forward fold, mountain pose, warrior 2, garland pose, bridge pose, and savasana.
Prithvi Mudra	: Bring the tip of ring finger to tip of thumb
Affirmation	: "I am safe, protected, and guided in this world."

Demo Video: Access "Root Chakra Practice" in your RECLAIMED Library: https://bit.ly/accesslibrary

SACRAL CHAKRA

Located in the lower abdomen, 2 inches below the navel and 2 inches in, this chakra represents...

- Our emotional body
- Our sensuality/sexuality
- Our capacity to go with the flow, to inspire connection and creativity
- To problem solve
- To empower our relationships

Suffice it to say, it is a hot spot for women, as there is so much *action* in this part of our bodies! If the sacral is unbalanced we may be feeling stuck, uninspired, disconnected, numb, immobilized, and isolated. It may manifest ...

In the body as:

- Chronic lower back pain
- Hip and pelvic issues
- Sexual and reproductive health challenges
- Urinary difficulties and kidney problems
- Too much energy flowing throughout the body

In the mind and heart as:

- Feeling emotionally amped up
- Feeling an emptiness and dissatisfaction with life
- Lacking self-control
- Seeking fulfillment outside of self, leading to extreme self-soothing behaviors and addictions
- Having an inability to cope, to problem solve
- Lacking creativity
- Having co-dependent relationships
- Detaching from self

Element	: Water
Color	: Orange
Pranayama	: Ujjayi
Movement Focus	: Pelvis and hips. Postures such as low lunge, half splits, goddess pose, wide-legged standing forward fold, exalted warrior, camel pose, locust or bow pose, and reclined bound angle pose.
Varuna Mudra	: Touch pad of little finger to pad of thumb
Affirmation	: "I am radiant, beautiful, creative, and enjoy a healthy and passionate life."

> **TRANSFORMATIONAL INSIGHT:** An unbalanced sacral chakra tends to manifest in the form of extreme self-soothing and addiction. If you are struggling in this regard, kindly, without judgement, observe your choices and behaviors. Remind yourself addictions can be subtle or significant, and we all have them, so dig deep here. Make a little list, not to call yourself out, but rather to sit in awareness. Restoring balance to this chakra through deeper connection, pranayama, movement, and mindfulness, can invite choices and behaviors that serve us far more constructively.

▶ **Demo Video:** Access "Sacral Chakra Practice" in your RECLAIMED Library: https://bit.ly/accesslibrary

SOLAR PLEXUS CHAKRA

Located in the upper abdomen, this chakra is at the heart of our identity and reflects personal power, passion, confidence, self-worth, self-responsibility, feeling in control of our lives, and overcoming fear. When in balance, it allows us to shine effervescently, with authenticity, confidence, and capacity. If it is burning too hot, feelings of insecurity, frustration, and anger can percolate... not hot enough, we may feel purposeless, lethargic, with no drive or desire. Imbalance may manifest...

In the body as:

- Chronic exhaustion
- Digestive problems
- Pancreatic or gall bladder issues

In the heart and mind as:

- Frustration
- Anger
- Aggression
- Stubbornness
- Judgment
- A controlling attitude
- Lack of confidence
- Self-esteem issues
- Self-criticism
- Rejection of fears
- Indecision
- Projection of responsibility
- Helplessness
- Loss of purpose
- Martyrdom

Element	: Fire
Color	: Yellow
Movement Focus	: To stoke the fire and support digestion use a core and detoxifying twist practice, inclusive of back bends to build energy and vigor. To cool your solar plexus jets use calming movements and breath: forward folds, moon salutations, extended exhalation, and alternate nostril breathing.
Pranayama	: Kapalabhati
Agni Mudra	: Fold the ring finger to the base of the thumb, and press with the thumb at the second phalange, hold the rest of the fingers straight.

Affirmation : "I live my life passionately, creatively, and with purpose."

> **TRANSFORMATIONAL INSIGHT:** When the third chakra is feeling balanced one experiences both respect and compassion for self.

HEART CHAKRA

Located in the center of the chest, above the heart, this chakra is about...

- Our ability to give and receive love, at its very best, unconditionally
- Setting healthy boundaries
- Cultivating compassion, contentment, joy, inner peace, and healthy ego

Imbalance may manifest...

In the body as:

- Asthma
- Wrist and arm discomfort/pain
- Shoulder and upper back issues
- Heart disease
- Breast cancer

In the heart and mind as:

- Codependency
- Fear of being alone
- Self-neglect
- Loss of identity
- Lack of boundaries
- A Yes-person at the expense of self
- Over-loving and over-giving to others
- Inability to receive generosity and love from others

TRANSFORMATIONAL INSIGHT: At its extreme of imbalance, one may experience detachment, isolation, lack of empathy, jealousy, resentment, and an inability to forgive. In its highest resonance, one feels authentic joy, gratitude, compassion, and love, for self and others.

Element   : Air
Color   : Green
Pranayama   : Bee Breath
Movement Focus : Back bending to emphasize kind opening of the front body, namely the chest and shoulders, while focusing on expansion, cultivating contentment, and compassion for self and others. Exploring postures such as cow-cat, cobra pose, upward-facing dog, puppy pose, warrior 1 with heart-opening backbend, fish pose, bridge pose, and reclined bound angle.

Lotus Mudra : Bring the base of your hands together at heart center... connect your pinkies to your thumbs... gently open the other fingers like a lotus blossoming. Emanate and receive love.

Affirmation : "I am love in all that I do."

It is also important to note when working to open shoulders, chest, and specifically the heart, that we go slowly, compassionately, and lovingly. Nudging the edges versus cracking the heart wide open, so to speak. If we are not yet in a state of readiness to receive, this can feel way too much and emotionally overwhelming. The emphasis here is on kind expansion.

Now, I am going to take a bit of a *chakra time out* to share with you a client case study specific to the Heart Chakra, following which we will return to our chakra exploration.

Client Case Study – Healing Her Torn Heart

This case study illustrates the power of perceiving our beings from an energetic standpoint, from the perspective of the chakras. When I completed my 500-hour teacher training in yoga therapy, part of the course work was submitting a paper to reflect our capacity to apply yoga to a specific manifestation of unwellness, be it physical and/or mental-emotional. I chose the topic of Yoga and Breast Cancer. Little did I know then that this project was preparing me to support one of my very first clients as a Yoga Therapist. I will call her Jane.

Jane was referred to me by one of my other wonderful clients. She was in recovery from her second round of breast cancer treatment, following a lengthy remission. Her cancer was back, and she was devastated.

A little background on Jane:

- In mid-50's
- A wife
- A mother of two boys, one in university and the other completing his last year of high school
- A daughter and care-giver for mom (mid-70's) in early stages of dementia
- Father deceased
- Two siblings, married with children, living in other countries
- Dog owner

- Self-identified Type 'A' Personality
- Senior executive at a Fortune 500 company

Jane felt she had been doing all the right things, and yet found herself battling once more. It was her desire for a different approach that led her to me. I began by helping Jane see herself as a whole being, comprised of breath, body, mind, energy, and soul. Together we structured a yoga and self-care strategy grounded in the Three Pillars of Pain-Free Living that addressed each of these integral layers. Our plan included:

- Soothing pranayama to encourage optimal breath and life force flow
- Restorative yoga practices to calm the nervous system and support lymphatic drainage
- Daily mindfulness and meditation to nourish awareness and foster connection to self and present moment
- Chakra exploration, with particular focus on an unbalanced heart chakra and its high correlation with breast cancer in women
- Deep soul work to re-align jane with her passion, purpose, and truth, and to re-ignite her servant's heart

All the above really resonated with Jane, and was instrumental in her healing journey, but it was our discussions around the heart chakra that yielded the most meaningful insights for her, relative to how she arrived energetically in her state of unwellness and how, through intentional living, she could shift her energy, restore balance, and empower her wellness.

As I mentioned, an unbalanced heart chakra has been shown scientifically to have a high correlation with the prevalence of breast cancer in women. Why? Well, look at Jane, wearing all the hats... wife... mom... daughter... caregiver... career woman... and doing it all to the nth degree, leaving her with little to no space for herself. One of our greatest *superpowers* as women is our capacity to nurture and nourish, provided we concurrently extend the same courtesy to ourselves. What happens instead? We become masters of showing up for others... partners... kids... parents... friends... work... pets... not necessarily in the order. We leave ourselves behind. We give love and serve at our own expense, neglecting our own needs and desires, and over time creating a deficit. A deficit that eventually leaves us feeling empty, resentful, unworthy and, at its most extreme, manifesting as discomfort, pain, and disease.

If we recall from our heart chakra conversation, it reflects our capacity to give and receive love, and women tend to be really good at the giving part, and not so much at the receiving part. Left unattended and perpetuated, this can leave us with a broken heart or, what is otherwise known as, a *torn heart chakra*. It is this tear that become insidious, inviting illness, more specifically, breast cancer which now commands our attention.

In Jane's case, we took time to explore the various roles in her life, identifying priorities and setting healthy boundaries relative to each relationship, recognizing that boundaries are profound acts of love for self and others. With renewed clarity and a commitment to serving self, Jane began the practice of courageously and compassionately speaking her truth... Throat Chakra... to bring balance to her relationships, to honor and heal her heart, to reclaim her life.

- Jane has been cancer-free for 7 years.
- She and her husband are happy empty nesters.
- She continues to lovingly support her mom.
- She is joyfully nearing retirement.
- She is now a restorative yoga teacher, supporting others in their healing journey.

THROAT CHAKRA

Located in the throat... surprise! Ha-ha! This chakra is about...

- Speaking our truth with authenticity, clarity, and confidence
- Articulating healthy boundaries kindly and compassionately
- Expressing creativity and freedom of spirit aligned with our heart's purpose

Imbalance may manifest...

In the body as:

- A sore throat
- An ear infection
- An imbalanced thyroid
- Neck and shoulder issues

In the heart and mind as:

- Poor listening skills
- Lacking boundaries
- Gossiping
- Being critical of others
- An inflated ego
- Patronizing attitude
- Ignorance
- Shyness
- Introversion

- Insecurity
- Fear of being out of control
- Fear of speaking your truth
- An inability to articulate boundaries
- Feeling and acting small
- Wearing your invisibility cloak

Element : Ether

Color : Blue

Pranayama : Bee Breath to stimulate the voice box, and to enlist both the active and cognitive senses of the throat, speech, and hearing. A little homework...Google Lion's Breath for a playful 6th chakra exploration... makes me smile just thinking of it!

Movement Focus : Neck and throat openers, such as neck rolls, reverse table, reverse plank, bridge pose, and fish pose.

Akasha Mudra : Touch the tip of the middle finger to the tip of the thumb. Morning is best for this mudra. Hold up to 45 minutes.

Affirmation : "I set and speak my boundaries, as an act of love and service to both self and others."

TRANSFORMATIONAL INSIGHT: When it comes to throat chakra, listening is just as important as speaking.

THIRD EYE CHAKRA

Located in the middle of the forehead between the eyebrows, this chakra is our center of command and reflects...

- Intuition
- Wisdom
- Clarity
- Decision-making
- Focus
- Concentration

It goes beyond ego.

Imbalance may manifest...

In the body as:

- Sinus problems
- Headaches
- Vision issues

In the heart and mind as:

- Overthinking
- Paralysis by analysis
- Feeling overwhelmed
- Anxiety
- Daydreaming
- Living in a fog
- Inability to concentrate
- Being distracted

- Moodiness
- Fear of the unknown
- Living too much in the future
- Feeling stuck in the past
- Inability to live in the present moment
- Disconnection from intuition
- Being unable to see yourself as you are
- Stubbornness

Element   : Light
Color   : Indigo or Purple
Pranayama   : Alternate Nostril Breathing
Movement Focus : All Seeing Slow Flow, with emphasis upon awareness, intuition, clarity, connection, mindfulness, and intention. Postures may include child's pose, puppy pose, dolphin pose, forearm plank, eagle pose.
Hakini Mudra   : Place all the fingertips together, you may wish to bring index fingers to rest gently at third eye
Affirmation   : "I see that I am connected to everything and everyone."

> **TRANSFORMATIONAL INSIGHT:** There is something to be said for a "woman's intuition". In fact, I believe it is one of our *superpowers*. However, over time, through distraction and societal narrative, we disconnect from our inner knowing. We begin to mistrust; we yield to external forces and the constant din of white noise. It's time for you to reclaim your keen and innate wisdom. You have magic in you!

CROWN CHAKRA

Yep, you guessed it, located at the crown of the head. It is where...

- Individual consciousness meets universal consciousness
- Spiritual transformation is possible
- We truly understand we are beyond self, and part of a bigger whole

At this point, our experience moves beyond our physical being and imbalance manifests more in our less tangible soulful being. It may manifest...

In the heart and mind as:

- Disenchantment
- Indifference
- Inflated ego
- Feeling above others
- Head in the clouds
- Detachment from body and earth experience
- Feeling uninspired
- Greed
- Mental muddiness

Element   : None
Color   : Violet or White
Pranayama   : Alternate Nostril Breathing or Kapalbhati

Movement Focus	: Inversions, anything that brings the crown of head toward or to the floor, such as standing forward fold, downward dog, rabbit pose, fish pose, supported headstand
Mudra of a Thousand Petals	: Place the tips of your index fingers and thumbs together to touch... palms open and away from you, forming a pyramid shape... allowing the remaining fingers to extend upward, keeping them straight. Raise this mudra to about 6 to 7 inches above the crown of your head. If there is any discomfort through shoulders and neck, work in the range of motion that feels just right for you
Affirmation	: "I am here to serve a purpose greater than myself."

TRANSFORMATIONAL INSIGHT: The crown chakra is also referred to as the Thousand Petal Lotus (simply love this visual!) and is the most subtle of the chakras, embodying pure consciousness and connection. When in balance, we enjoy an unwavering faith in our intuitive capacity for optimal living.

TO RECAP:

- ✓ You have been introduced to your subtle body, the chakra system, that in essence sheaths your physical body. And yes, we have just scratched the surface here!

- ✓ You now know, without doubt, that you are an energetic entity.

- ✓ You have learned that the chakras, overactive or underactive, may be balanced through breath, kind movement, mindfulness, meditation, mudra, and affirmation.

- ✓ Take a little time to reflect upon the chakras, as they relate back to the 3 Pillars of Pain-Free Living. Feel free to journal out your insights to fortify your knowledge and understanding.

- ✓ You now have another doorway, another opportunity to keep honing awareness, deepening connection, and taking mindful, purposeful action.

- ✓ YOU ARE LEARNING TO MAKE A DAILY HABIT OF BALANCING YOUR ENERGETIC BLUEPRINT.

Are you ready to start *Rockin' Your Chakras*? Of course, you are!

Where do we go next?

In **Chapter 8: Magical Mindfulness**, we go intentionally inward to strengthen our powers of observation, so that we may invite stillness and create space for clarity and deeper connection. This, in turn, allows us to step confidently into aligned action and to impel optimal and enduring progress and growth. How about we throw a little prevention in there for good measure? Think accessible, doable mindfulness and meditation practices that support your Three Pillars of Pain-Free Living and serve to open yet another doorway through which you may move to actualize your sustainable whole health healing and recovery. Meet you there!

CHAPTER 8

Magical Mindfulness

Take time each day to slow down...
to settle into stillness... to go inward.

Breathe... listen... feel.

Play... explore... notice.

Nudge edges, adjust, align.

Give yourself what you need, so you may be
the very best version of you,

in any given moment.

The practice of meditation can be perceived as overwhelming, and trust me when I say, "I get it!" If you had told me ten years ago that I would be sitting in stillness or as close to stillness as I can get, from 5-15-25 minutes, observing my thoughts and letting them be as they are, I would have said, "You are crazy, no freaking way!" Now, I welcome the opportunity to do so. Like everything else, it has been a practice. I did not get here overnight. I would also suggest that activities, like your asana practice, walking, running, and cycling, can also be powerful forms of *moving meditation* and a great place to begin your mindfulness practice. If you are ready to settle into a more traditional meditation, find a quiet place and get comfortable, preferably seated, to avoid falling asleep. If you do, who cares. You probably need it! Settle into stillness as best as you can. If you need to make an adjustment throughout your meditation, do so, it's OK. Close your eyes, if this feels right for you, or keep them open, maybe even set your gaze on a lit candle to support your focus. This steady gaze in yoga is called *drishti*. Start with 3-5 minutes... no pressure. Set a timer if needed, increasing duration as you feel comfortable. What do you do? You notice, that's all, nothing more, nothing less. You do not need to empty your mind and think nothing, but rather observe the thoughts as they percolate for you... no judgement... no need to do anything with them... just observe and let them go. If the same thought rises for you again... notice it... no judgement... no action required... once again, set it adrift... let your thoughts come... let your thoughts go.

Meditation can bring much-needed clarity, a reprieve from the stranglehold of negative inner dialogue. It can slow things down physically, mentally, emotionally, energetically, and soulfully. It can empower you to sit safely with your thoughts, leaving your concerns feeling smaller and more manageable, and leaving you feeling stronger, more at ease.

Meditation is thus another great tool in your self-care arsenal. There are lots of great apps out there to support your meditation exploration. All that is required, on your part, is an open mind and an open heart.

FOSTERING A MINDFULNESS PRACTICE

So, where to begin? If mindfulness practice is new to you, it can be helpful to start with a guided meditation that offers vocal cues and touchpoints throughout to support your capacity to breathe and be in the present moment. Monkey-mind is a real thing, gang, and sometimes we need a little help to quell the mental mayhem! One such way to do this is through a Guided Body Scan. This technique allows you to explore mindfulness relative to sensation, feeling, and experience within your physical body. It invites tangibility, in that you remain *in body*, feeling grounded, safe, and supported by the earth beneath you. What else might it gift you? Let's find out.

GUIDED BODY SCAN

Practicing a body scan on a regular basis has many powerful benefits. It...

- Brings focus to your mind
- Shifts your attention away from negative thoughts
- Reduces anxiety
- Reduces stress
- Deepens connection between mind and body

Are you ready to give it a try? Awesome!

Audio Recording: Access "Guided Body Scan" in your RECLAIMED Library: https://bit.ly/accesslibrary

YOGA NIDRA

This form of guided meditation became my *go-to* when I was in recovery from acute anxiety. Literally, I did it day and night, whenever needed, and it made all the difference. What is it exactly?

Yogic sleep, as it is commonly known, is an immensely powerful meditation technique, and is one of the easiest yoga practices to develop and maintain. It starts with a body scan and then flows into a deep visualization. Often, it is specifically themed to support a particular aspect of healing. For example, there are Yoga Nidras for sleep, chronic physical and or mental-emotional pain, fears and limiting beliefs, the list goes on.

TRANSFORMATIONAL INSIGHT:
1 Hour of Yoga Nidra = 4 Hours of Deep Sleep

PRACTICE TIPS:

1. You can do a Yoga Nidra at any point in your day, but ideally, it can be wonderful to do before bed. You can just drift off into la-la land. It also comes in handy if you wake in the middle of the night and have difficulty falling back asleep. I have woken many a morning with a headset on!

2. Finding the right Nidra for you is key. You may or may not resonate with a particular voice, this is normal. Seek an experience that allows you to be as fully present, as still as possible, without distraction. There are many options to explore out there in cosmic cyberspace. When exploring on-line, take the time to find themes and offerings that truly resonate with you.

3. The intention is not to fall asleep in Yoga Nidra, but rather to find yourself floating in the *sweet spot* between consciousness and unconsciousness. And if you fall asleep, it's OK, you obviously needed the rest. So, enjoy it!

4. Find a place (maybe bed) where you may lie very comfortably, supporting your body with pillows and blankets as required. Make sure you are cozy, as your body temperature will drop as the Nidra progresses.

5. Be as comfortable as possible. This helps you remain as still as possible throughout the Nidra. And, if you have a *nose-tickle*, attend to it. Hold space for the perfectly-imperfect!

6. As with all else, it takes practice to be present and surrender to the process. Be sure to be kind, patient, and compassionate with yourself.

Yoga Nidra has been positively transformative for my clients and may contribute significantly to calming your nervous system, inviting ease, healing, and a sense of restfulness to both your mind and body. Tuck this one away in your easy access toolkit and have fun exploring!

Audio Recording: Access "Yoga Nidra" in your RECLAIMED Library: https://bit.ly/accesslibrary

TO RECAP:

✓ Meditation and mindfulness are two of the fundamental ways we can begin to empower a day-to-day, moment-to-moment habit of Authentic Awareness (First Pillar).

✓ Meditation does not need to be hard or go on forever. Nor does it require you to empty your head, levitate, or leave your body.

✓ It does encourage you to be present, aware, connected, and receptive.

- ✓ It does inspire greater focus, clarity, and aligned action which supports capacity, growth, and sustainable transformation.

- ✓ A Guided Body Scan can be a great introduction to meditation and mindfulness, as it serves as a trusted bridge between your physical and mental states of being.

- ✓ Yoga Nidra is a powerful guided meditation, a game-changer when it comes to calming the nervous system, alleviating pain, and supporting sleep challenges.

- ✓ Take a little time to reflect upon what you have learned in this chapter, as it relates back to the Three Pillars of Pain-Free Living. Feel free to journal out your insights to fortify your knowledge and understanding.

- ✓ You now have another doorway, another opportunity to keep honing awareness, deepening connection, and taking mindful, purposeful action.

- ✓ YOU ARE LEARNING TO MAKE A DAILY HABIT OF MINDFULNESS.

My hope is that you are now feeling magically mindful, and with each passing chapter you are cranking up your toolkit and stepping more fully into your capacity for *feel-good living*.

Often, one of the challenges of going inward, is coming face to face with your limiting beliefs and fears. But doing so is necessary. Why? It is these same limiting beliefs and fears that tend to immobilize you, hold you back, and keep you stuck. In **Chapter 9: EmBOLDened Fear**, you learn how to engage with your fear, kindly, compassionately, courageously, patiently, and lovingly, so you can break through the self-imposed barriers and set yourself free! This is honestly one of my most favorite subjects as, in many ways, it is the master key to the robust reclamation of our lives!

Now, affirm for yourself, "I am not fearless, but I am brave."

Let's do this, together.

"For me, meditation has always felt out of reach and impossible, the idea of settling into any form of stillness, uncomfortable and overwhelming. Being introduced to the Guided Body Scan has opened up my mind to the value of slowing down and making it feel accessible. The practice is not long, which I like, and brings a comforting, present moment tangibility... a welcome ease. It allows me to perceive my physical body through different eyes and to connect more deeply to its day-to-day experience. It is fostering an enthusiasm and curiosity for meditation for the very first time."

– 1:1 Reclaimed Mastery Client

From Julie's Journal and Journey

Catch a ride on your truth trajectory
October 8th, 2018

I am here to serve. I am here to inspire. I am here to love.
I am here to live my truth.
- Deepak Chopra

Sounds like a pretty spectacular ride, doesn't it?! That's because it is. Take a moment... even if this exact moment of your life has you hanging out in darker places... to really ponder the extraordinary happenings in your life, present and past, personally, and professionally, the happenings that make the fire in your belly ignite, your skin tingle, your breath catch, and your heart skip a beat. I would like to suggest these experiences, the ones that literally rock your world, that feel like full-on spontaneous combustion and compel you forward as if you were possessed by mystical forces, are directly aligned with your core being and Your Fundamental Truth. It is in these cataclysmic moments when the real you is being called to action; Your Purpose is literally calling out to you and saying, "Hey, you, over here, this is where you are going to work your magic in the world, where you are going to make your difference. "Can you hear me?! Feel me?! See me?! This is who you are. For the love of Pete, please pay attention!"

And so, you do, for a little while, but life happens. It hurts, you get distracted, maybe you give way to others' expectations of you. Maybe you hurt people, maybe you were the one hurt. Maybe you suffered trauma. Maybe you self-soothe in less-than healthy ways. And yeah, maybe you find yourself feeling really freaking alone, set adrift on a swelling sea of self-destruction.

Now, tell me this, does some or all of this 'delightful' inner diatribe stuck on 'repeat', no less, sound familiar to you? "It's all my fault..., I blame myself for it all... I did this... I deserve to suffer... I am a failure.... I am not enough... I am worthless... I am useless... I must have done something really, really bad in my last life because karma is biting me in the ass this time." Whoa! Stop the presses! Say to yourself, "This is the quintessential quagmire of exaggeration and flat-out lies."

Firstly, you are not solely responsible for the suffering of the world. I know it feels like it some days, but you alone don't get to lay claim to this title.

Secondly, you do not exist in a bubble. You are in constant relationship with those around you, and guess what, they are making choices and decisions as well.

Thirdly, sometimes things simply happen in life, completely beyond your control, and there is absolutely nothing you could have done to prevent its occurrence. Do you take responsibility and own your part? Yes, but only your part. Read that again! Do you have a lesson to learn? Well, that's entirely up to you. If you do, you will make better, healthier choices. What's the 'cherry on top'? You invite perspective, acceptance, forgiveness, and freedom into your life.

As they say, "Live and learn." Do the work... get out of your own way... aim for authenticity... catch a ride on your truth trajectory... choose to re-connect with your passions and purpose... do this daily and deeply. This is who you are. Trust and have faith. It will lead you in the direction of integrity, wholeness, healing, and at long last, will set you free. Give flight to your dreams and desires and know with your whole heart that you are most deserving of living your life inspired.

CHAPTER 9

EmBOLDened Fear

take your deepest fear
wrap it in your arms
hold it tight
give it nothing but love
honor it
respect it
nudge its edges
kindly
compassionately
patiently
walk with it
move through it
receive growth
revel in release
this is the gift

In this chapter, we are going to go toe-to-toe, in the kindest of ways, with our fears and limiting beliefs. I can honestly tell you these are among my most favorite exercises to explore with my clients, where fear is emboldened, and where our greatest untapped potential is discovered and set free. It is the best treasure hunt upon which you will ever embark.

WHAT ARE LIMITING BELIEFS?

1. We create limiting beliefs because our less-than-stellar experiences and history have marked us with a sense of lack and vulnerability, and the story we create, based upon minimal evidence and maximal assumptions, becomes our truth.

2. If left unchecked, limiting beliefs amplify into a perceived threat, activating the fight-flight-freeze-fawn response, and serve to perpetuate a vicious cycle of unnecessary self-protection.

3. Over time, we cease to trust ourselves, negating our intuition, undermining our self-confidence, convincing ourselves that the answers we most desire are to be found elsewhere.

4. We keep searching. We keep repeating. We feel stuck... over, and over, again.

5. Limiting beliefs then become excuses and make us reliant on others and circumstances over which we have little or no control.

What's the alternative? We...

- Go inward.
- Meet the fear.
- Sit with it.
- Acknowledge it.
- Evaluate it.
- Build a relationship with it.
- Empower it.
- Learn to use fear to our advantage.

How are we going to do this? Well, you've got homework!

In this exercise you will:

1. Learn how to surrender your self-created fears, limiting beliefs, and obstacles to catapult yourself into your fullest potential. This process begins with the White Sheet Meditation.

2. Learn how to construct a healthy, positive relationship with fear, one that mobilizes you into mindful action, because not doing so, not leaning into your passion and purpose, is more painful than the fear itself.

3. Understand that fear is good. Fear matters. It means you care, and your passion and purpose are awakening.

4. Learn to meet your fear and use it to propel you forward, to amplify your life and your capacity.

5. Learn how to show up authentically, with confidence, in all the layers of your being, to own it.

WHITE SHEET MEDITATION

Audio Recording: Access "White Sheet Meditation" in your RECLAIMED Library: https://bit.ly/accesslibrary

1. Listen to the White Sheet Mediation.

2. Ensure you are in a quiet space with no distractions.

3. Make sure you have the time to listen to the meditation in its entirety.

4. Give yourself the grace to sit with everything that comes up for you during this meditation.

5. Afterwards, take out your journal and let all the words, feelings and ideas that bubbled up flow onto your paper.

6. Who was present for you at your four corners of the sheet? Who wasn't? Do you feel a newfound clarity relative to your support system?

7. What specific limiting beliefs and fears were gathered and set free? How did that feel for you in breath, body, mind, energy, and soul?

8. Don't hold back here, get all your limiting beliefs out, and think about what would be possible for you if those limiting beliefs did not exist.

9. Reflect upon how you may transform your fears into intentional, empowered action.

Hot Tip: This meditation is full of layers, subtle and not-so-subtle insights. I have had the greatest breakthroughs with clients who have moved through the meditation repeatedly. For example, different people, pets, and entities may appear at your four corners. Often new limiting beliefs and fears can be revealed and liberated.

"I am not fearless, but I am brave."

HOW DO WE STOP FEARING THE FEAR?

Compassionate Connection (Pillar Two) allows us to meet fear with grace, capacity, and courage. How so? Let's take a closer look.

When it comes to self-exposure:

Often, vulnerability is mistaken for fragility. But, in fact, our capacity to be vulnerable, to open our hearts and minds to the human experience takes, shall we say, big kahunas! The oh-so-sweet reward of doing this is *Authentic Loving and Living*.

Take a moment to reflect upon your inner demons, the ones that like to run amok between your heart and your head. Now, capture them with great care in the palm of your hand... they feel smaller here... more manageable. Remind yourself, you are not defined by your oh-so-sensitive extra special guests. They are simply pieces of you, yearning for your undivided attention, your respect, your compassion. Choose to see them... to hear them... to feel them... to hold them tighter... to love them harder... to mindfully move together towards greater self-understanding, self-acceptance, integration, wholeness, and healing. Invite integration.

When it comes to overcoming pain and healing a broken heart:

Pain, when denied, eventually manifests itself as an almighty sucker-punch, commanding your attention, and forcing you to deal with it. It demands that you sit in it... feel it deeply... process it fully... until, at long last, you may... settle into peace and set yourself free.

If, in your lifetime, you have successfully managed and moved through periods of depression and/or anxiety by making use of available resources, learned skills, and self-care practices, then you have developed resiliency. You have a history of healing and recovery. This is a very good thing and will serve you well should you find yourself immersed once more in a deep struggle. Gently remind yourself this is not your first rodeo. Trust in your capacity. You have done it before. You will do it again.

Let me ask you, what is your why? What is your impetus to heal, to recover, to do the really hard work? My why? I wish to become *The Very Best Me Possible*, grounded in my truth, stronger, more joyful, more loving. More freaking real! I am also bound and determined to set an example for my son, one that says, yes, this life can be damn hard, and yes, it can have us landing with an almighty "THUMP!" at rock bottom, leaving us feeling battered, bruised, and broken. However, it is more than possible to rise up, to live better, fully engaged, and emboldened.

Finding your voice and speaking your truth

Now, this demands the ultimate in bravery from you. Humans are master storytellers, and the stories you tell yourself, particularly when you are in a vulnerable mental-emotional state, can be epic masterpieces in fiction. When you are hurting deeply and/or feeling fearful you often get lost in unfair judgements of yourself and others, and you may make grossly inaccurate assumptions relative to your relationships and day to day experiences.

One of the keys to healing and recovery, is getting skilled at dealing in the facts and grounding yourself in healthy perspectives, not allowing yourself to fall victim to an imagination gone wild, relative to what you think you may see, hear, and feel, in any given moment. How do you make sure you are keeping it real? You slow it all down and ask yourself, "Is this a truth or is it an unfounded belief?" When necessary, you seek clarification from others to ensure you are responding fairly, compassionately, patiently, and from a place of honesty, integrity, and reality.

Now, let me ask...

Is it easy? Nope. It's really tough work. Does it get easier with practice? Big, enthusiastic, YES!

- Are you hiding behind surface smiles, veiled in masks and facades?

- Are you suffering in silence, afraid of sharing your vulnerabilities and speaking your truth?

- Are you fearful of hurting and/or disappointing others, perhaps of being judged and/or abandoned?

Do some, perhaps all of the above, hold you back from making key decisions and actively seeking the support your heart, mind, and body, so desperately desire and deserve?

If this is you, and you find yourself deeply struggling with life, and more specifically your mental health, just know, you are not alone. I would also like to gently encourage you to give yourself what you need, to choose to access the abundance of resources out there that could make all the difference to your healing, recovery, and well-being. Of course, it won't be easy, but if you persist, it will be worth it. And sadly, you may experience some judgement and a sense of abandonment along the way. This is not your work to do. Your priority is you. What I can tell you, your tried-and-trues will be right there, by your side. They are your very best cheerleaders and advocates, as you move through the good, the bad, and the ugly of your journey. Think of your White Sheet Meditation.

If you knew for sure that nudging this door open with the greatest of care and compassion, in a trusted place and space, resulted in your setting yourself free from the grips of unrelenting darkness and returned you to living your life inspired, would it not be worth it? I do know this, "You are worth it. What are you waiting for?"

Am I being honest with myself?

As part of my personal healing journey, I ask myself this question constantly, "What stories, little white lies, or whoppers, driven by... my fears, vulnerabilities, assumptions, and selfishness... do I tell myself to deny, deflect, and protect myself and others." I have absolutely done this, particularly to mask my mental health challenges, and I still catch myself doing it. I would suggest we all do, in varying degrees, at various times in our lives. Perhaps it's even in our DNA, part of our innate human drive to survive and thrive at all costs.

When I left the hospital almost four years ago, I had three goals:

1. Free myself from co-dependent relationships. To understand and own my part and to evolve healthier relationships.

2. Independence – mentally, emotionally, energetically, soulfully, and yes, financially. The capacity to know I can stand on my own two feet, regardless of relationship outcomes.

3. To honor, speak, and action my truth. To be real.

Moving towards and actualizing these goals, through daily and diligent practice, has required brutal, painful honesty on my part, and has been, without doubt, some of the most grueling work I have ever done...

- Humbling myself
- Holding myself accountable
- Rethinking and redirecting choices, actions, and behaviors
- Practicing more effective ways of being in the world
- Serving myself
- Serving others
- Striving to become the most authentic me possible.

Do I stumble? Yes. Am I getting better at it? Bigger YES. Let's face it, at the end of the day, it is I who must live and make peace with the consequences of my choices. And it is I who chooses to engage in an honest relationship with myself.

If you are going to live the life of your dreams, the life you deserve, then you must constantly be asking yourself, "Am I being truly honest with myself?"

The Gift of Befriending Your Fear

There are times when choosing courage can feel like you are going left while everybody else is going right, particularly when moving through the journey of bloody-hard-work-healing. And if you are being effective in your recovery, personal change for the better is inevitable and, not to mention, celebrated! In the spirit of transformation, you also begin to respond and behave differently, relative to your new truth, to the relationships in your life, to your new goals and dreams. All sounds awesome, right? And it is. However, for those around you, there may be fear, discomfort, mistrust, even anger, as you no longer react or engage as you once did or, more importantly, as they expect you to do. It becomes a what's-happening-here and what-do-I-do-with- it kind of exchange. It's not that your loved ones do not wish for you to heal, they absolutely do, but change for you means change for them, and they may not be comfortable or ready to meet you there or frankly even dislike our updated, upgraded (from our perspective) operating system. And guess what? That's okay. You, however, must continue to practice diligently, and to hold steady in your courageous, reconstructive life pursuits; You must ultimately come to trust yourself.

So, now that you have had the opportunity to befriend your limiting beliefs and fears, to distinguish between a fear that is truly a threat to your safety and one that is more a figment of an imagination run wild, and then to release unsubstantiated limiting beliefs, what's next? Well, this is the fun part, you are going to write a love letter to yourself! Yep, for real!

MANIFESTATION AND LOVE NOTE TO SELF

What you will need:

- Courageous heart and open mind

- Journal and pen

- Envelope and sheet(s) of paper

- Access "One Year from Now Visualization Exercise" in your RECLAIMED Library: https://bit.ly/accesslibrary.

Visualization Exercise:

1. Choose a time w\hen you will not be interrupted.

2. Create your Visualization Space:

   - Find a peaceful place with a table and comfortable chair.

   - Your computer is on the table, with the "One Year from Now Visualization Exercise" open so you can comfortably access after each visualization step.

   - Work at your own pace. This doesn't have to be done in one sitting. Create a schedule once you get a feel for the process.

   - You may wish to have calming music in the background.

3. Download "ONE YEAR FROM NOW VISUALIZATION EXERCISE" from your RECLAIMED Library: https://bit.ly/accesslibrary

4. In the space provided on the first row of your chart, put your name and then insert a fab picture of yourself in the space provided.

5. Review the MY VISUALIZATION PROMPTS listed in the first column. They are also listed below. Some may not resonate/ fit for you and that's OK. They are not obligatory. However, they may bring up some interesting thoughts which you might want to jot down... or not. The visualizations have their own energy, and some will take more time than others. Just go with the flow. What do you envision for yourself One Year from Today? MY VISUALIZATION PROMPTS include...

- The space where I am living.
- How I am feeling emotionally.
- How I am feeling physically.
- How I am feeling spiritually.
- What people experience in my presence.
- The things I am doing to have fun in my life.
- The things I am doing to celebrate myself.
- What I am doing to support myself financially.
- What I am doing to shift my view of spending money to one where less is more.
- The quality of my relationship with _____ (insert name and insert additional rows for the other relationships you wish to visualize).
- What I am doing in my community to reduce social

inequalities.

- What I am doing in my home and community to heal the environment.
- What I am doing to increase my involvement in community decision-making.
- Anything else that comes to mind.

6. Visualization will connect you more deeply to your Third Eye (mid-forehead, between brows), as we talked about earlier in Rock Your Chakras. This is the place within you that reflects wisdom, insight, intuition, and manifestation. This exploration is about seeing and energizing what it is you would like to see unfold for yourself, in every layer of your being...in your relationships with self and others... in your work life, in your community... with Mother Earth, herself. It's about freeing yourself from limiting beliefs, fears, pain, and reclaiming your life in every possible way.

So, really reflecting and thinking about where you want to be in all those aspects of your life, journal out the following in the space provided on the chart.

- Where do you see yourself?
- What do you wish to be doing?
- What actions are you taking?
- With whom do you want to be engaging?

Think about your key relationships.

- What do they look like?
- Feel like?

- How are they healthier?
- Invigorated?
- Revitalized?

See yourself whole. And, One Year from Today, what is your highest vision for yourself?

NEXT STEPS

1. You are now going to draft a letter to yourself. It will literally start with "Dear _____" (insert your name), and will encompass what that vision is for yourself, identifying your goals and manifesting your desired reality, connecting deeply to wisdom, to insight, to that Third Eye Space, which I like to refer to as your Personal Intuition Portal, PIP for short! Take time with this, don't rush it. Visualize exactly the 'Who, What, Where, When, Why, and How' about everything you wish for yourself One Year from Today.

2. You are going to write it all out in a kind, beautiful Love Letter to Yourself. As fully as you can see it, colorfully and vividly. Envision yourself stepping into this optimal state of being, regardless of whether life is presenting challenges a year from now, or not. Just remember 'perfectly imperfect' is enough. What will have shifted is your capacity to meet it, to show up in that space, from a place of grace and equanimity.

3. Once you have completed your love letter, you are going to fold it up, put it in the envelope, seal it, write the 'One Year from Today' date on it, and tuck it away in a safe place.

4. Create an event in your calendar as reminder to retrieve and read your Love Letter to Myself. Be sure to include the location of envelope!

5. Have fun with this! Be honest with yourself, stretch yourself, but keep it achievable, i.e., marrying Brad Pitt or Gal Gadot is likely not in the cards, no matter how much you manifest! Continue to embrace and energize your manifestation over the next 365 days. Make it a daily habit.

6. When you return to it one year from now, do this with an open mind and heart. See your growth and transformation and perhaps some of the struggles that remain. This is your opportunity to observe and celebrate your journey.

So, settle into the writing, enjoy the process and envisioning what you deeply desire for your future, and what you are ultimately working towards, as you see yourself whole and heal yourself whole.

TO RECAP:

✓ You examined limiting beliefs and fear, from the place of Authentic Awareness (Pillar One), and how to discern between real threat to personal safety, and perceived threat based upon past, negative experience, and assumption.

✓ Through Compassionate Connection (Pillar 2) you got cozy with your perceived fears, acknowledging their presence, appreciating their message, and choosing to utilize them as an impetus for growth, and getting out of your own way.

✓ You learned how to surrender self-created fears, limiting beliefs, and obstacles, to take Aligned Action (Pillar 3) towards manifesting your highest vision possible and actualizing your full human potential.

✓ Oh! And you discovered you are in possession of your very own PIP, your Personal Intuition Portal!

✓ As always, take a little time to reflect upon what you have learned in this chapter, as it relates back to the Three Pillars of Pain-Free Living. Feel free to journal out your insights to fortify your knowledge and understanding.

✓ You now have, yet another doorway, another opportunity to keep honing awareness, deepening connection, and taking mindful, purposeful action.

Is your bravery muscle feeling flexed? Do you see that you are stronger and more courageous than you ever imagined possible? Can you choose to trust and believe THIS IS WHO YOU ARE? Because you can. Take a moment to celebrate this levelling up in your capacity!

Where do you go from here? Well, to what I believe is the integration piece of this puzzle, to what brings all the above together, and offers a cohesive infrastructure, a rich web of connection, from which you may embrace the profound gifts and challenges of living in relationship with the earth, with yourself, with others, and in global community. Any guesses? Drumroll, please.

Next, we will be diving, heart first into **Chapter 10: Becoming a Gratitude Mindset Expert.**

Life Happens to Us All

How do we find the bliss in our becoming?

We choose it.

We choose intention.

We choose perfectly imperfect.

We choose compassion.

We choose to wonder, to keep our hearts and minds wide open.

We choose to feel both the light and the darkness.

We choose to keep going, to embrace the bittersweet bliss of being.

In this place.

In this space.

In this time.

We choose to leave a legacy that ripples and resonates, graciously, infinitely, beyond our last breath.

We choose.

"The White Sheet Meditation is incredibly powerful, multi-layered, and full of surprises. I return to it over and over again, when I am feeling overwhelmed by my fears and pain. It connects me energetically to my support system, and helps me see, hear, feel, and safely release my discomforts. I feel both courage and love settle into the space created in the letting go."

- Reclaimed Mastery Client

"I must tell you that the process of honing in on sacrosanct values and creating this manifesto has been wholly transformative, my sweet-souled coach. Through them, I already find myself course correcting relative to my depressive tendencies. Beyond huge. So much love coming your way for shining this light!!!!!!!"

- RECLAIMED Mastery Client

From Julie's Journal and Journey

The masks we wear
June 4, 2019

I would like to suggest that most of us move through our lives donning the necessary masks to fit in, to find acceptance, and to create the illusion that life is indeed the best thing ever.

I am going to share a little story here. I moved from Thunder Bay, Ontario, small town living, relatively speaking, to London, Ontario. This was the beginning of my Grade 11th year. Enter traumatic life event! Thunder Bay was home to me, where I had the world by the balls. I was top of my class academically, one of the top female athletes in the city. I had a best friend... we were known as the *Dynamic Duo* for the magic we created together on the basketball and volleyball courts. I had a great group of friends. And I was dating our school's senior football quarterback. Life was good... or so it seemed.

Fast forward to the first day of school in London. My mom pulls up to the school, that we already know is populated like a small city, and the very first words out of my mouth are, "This looks more like a correctional facility than a school!" I am dying! As I recall, my sister pops effervescently out of the car. She is braver than me, excited to start Grade 9, and the world is her oyster. I don't move.

Mom says, "OK, Jules, you got this! In you go!"

Me, one of the most compliant people I know, says, "No. I am not going in there."

Mom says, "But all of your new friends are in there, waiting to meet you."

Me, silently, says, "Yeah, I'm onto you, Mom. Reverse psychology is not going to work here."

Me, out loud, says, "No."

Mom says, "OK, there is a mall across the street. Let's go get you a special back-to-school-outfit and then you go in. Deal?"

Me, "Deal."

An hour or so later, I enter this said correctional facility, dressed in a white teddy bear blouse and a jean skirt, and, of course, my big, rocking, 80's hair... ha! ha!

Looking back, I am well aware, it was here I came to create and perfect my wardrobe of masks. During the first six months, paralyzing shyness had me eating lunch in my math room, for crying out loud, the cafeteria was like a small village itself, and, over the year I became known as "The Girl Who Smiles a Lot." I did this because I didn't want people to think I was a snob.

And thank goodness, for sport. This was the only time I felt I was truly me, shining on the basketball and volleyball court, and Fosbury Flopping over a high jump bar. Here I belonged. I made a difference. Here I had value. And here I could lead. To this day, I thank my lucky stars for my athletic endeavors, my awesome teammates, and my kick-ass coaches. I was drowning. They saved me.

Now, allow me to introduce The Many Masks of Julie, circa 80's & 90's. There was...

Star Student Julie... Star Athlete Julie... Perfectionist Julie... Fat Julie... Skinny Julie...Pretty Julie... Ugly Julie... Loved Julie... Hated Julie... Bulimic Julie... Anorexic Julie... Over-Exerciser Julie... Never Enough Julie... Useless Julie... Painfully Shy Julie... Socially Inept Julie... Smiling Julie... Empath Julie... Introvert Julie... Depressed Julie... Happy Julie... Sensitive Julie... Strong Julie... Vulnerable Julie... Shameful Julie... Worthless Julie... Exhausted Julie... Suicidal Julie... Survivor Julie.

And by no means, is this list exhaustive, but I don't want to overwhelm you- ha! ha! Heck, I could have used a Full-Time Personal Assistant to look after all of those Julies! From eleven to twenty years of age, I was completely lost in myself. It has taken me literally a lifetime of battling eating disorders, depression, and five suicide attempts to finally unveil, deconstruct, reconstruct, find, and fall madly in love with myself... as I am. Yes, I have come a long way, but I continue to journey resolutely in the pursuit of full healing and recovery. Mental health management is a daily, diligent practice in self-care. For me, this includes a small-but-mighty trusted tribe and a keen commitment to diet, sleep, yoga, meditation, breath-work, walking, counselling, and the right medication for me.

Somewhere along the line... and I am going to suggest men get the even-shorter-end-of-the-stick on this one... we learn to hide our true feelings, to buck up, and pretend all is A-OK, no problem, nothing to see here. It's absolutely, bloody freaking perfect! All of this, in the name of acceptance and belonging. Note: There is nothing healthy about this, for any of us!

Unveiling takes tremendous courage. It takes trust in self and others... it takes compassion and patience... and it takes oodles of practice. So, how 'bout we all just decide to get real and stop pretending? Let's, collectively, choose to be honest, and to walk through the good stuff and the heart-shattering stuff together. No more throwing masks on to hide our truths, our hurts, losses, and disappointments. Rather, revealing our genuine selves and showing up authentically for each other; sharing stories, friendship, connection, and community.

I will leave you with this quote by Megan Devine, grief advocate and author. It is the title of one of her books...

"It's OK that You're Not OK."

The sooner we collectively realize this, the sooner we set ourselves free, and get on with living an authentic life.

Today, and moving forward, I wish you the freedom to be really you. I wish you profound connection with self and with others. We are stronger together.

CHAPTER 10

Becoming a Gratitude Mindset Expert

Before my mental health crisis and subsequent suicide attempt in late 2017, I was known as *The Girl with The Pink-Colored Glasses*. I could see the possibility in everything, and my capacity for hope was infinite. It was always figureoutable. I was counted upon for my creative problem-solving and was often heard saying, "It will be fine." Solutions were my expertise and, honestly, I loved the challenge. Not only that, but I was also renowned for the way I passionately and consistently lived from a place of deep gratitude.

When life imploded and I found myself sucker-punched, yet again, by depression, suffice it to say, there were no more pretty shades of pink. In fact, there was not a single glimmer of light. The fall was hard and fast, beyond rock bottom, and I had lost all will to go on... hope extinguished... gratitude snuffed out.

So, how did I get from there to here... writing this book... talking about gratitude... championing life once more? I am not going to lie. It has been bloody hard work. Growth and healing have presented themselves in many forms over the past few years, including hospital stays, counselling, support from family, friends, and community, and what, I like to call, a very 'conscious unveiling'. I credit three things for saving my life: daily yoga, walking, and gratitude practice.

Quick side note: Those who know me, will have heard me champion the statement, "It's all yoga." Relationships... eating... self-care... walking... gratitude... are all great examples of what I refer to as "Our Off the Mat Practice" where the magic really happens.

Introducing what I like to call the 3 A's of Gratitude...

- Attitude
- Acceptance
- Action

ATTITUDE

Gratitude is a mindset, a mindful, conscious choice, a daily practice... just as choosing to eat healthy food or not... moving our bodies or not...surrounding ourselves with nourishing relationships or not... choosing to be grateful...or not... are all mindsets We are all familiar with the Tony Robbins' quote, "Where focus goes, energy flows."

So, how do you cultivate a Daily Gratitude Mindset?

You begin the moment your eyes open... before you reach for your phone... before you hit the ground running to get that first sip of coffee. Traditionally, we think of yoga as arriving upon our mat for a scheduled class, to breathe, and to move in our bodies. But, in fact, our yoga practice begins the moment we wake, the first moment we return our conscious awareness to breathing, physical sensation, and emotions... taking time to nudge edges... a little stretch here... a little stretch there... gathering insights... embracing our aliveness and celebrating it. Now, replace the word 'yoga' with 'gratitude.' Bring your conscious awareness immediately to those things for which you are grateful, receiving the gifts of simply breathing and being.

Here is a simple exercise you may be practicing already. Keep a Gratitude Journal at your bedside. Upon completing your short but sweet morning mind, body, soul inventory, write down, at minimum, one thing for which you are grateful. For some of us, depending on where we are at and what we are currently moving through in life, one thing can be a struggle to find. I have been there, and I get it. But commit to yourself to squeak one out. It does not have to be larger than life. It could be simply waking to the song of birds at your window... your morning cup of tea and the comfort it brings... the feeling of being ensconced in your cozy blankets. As you continue to practice and build confidence, aim for two, three, five things for which you are grateful... right now... in present moment. Write them out and then read them out loud... hear yourself speak these words... all this before you do anything else.

And just before bed... you guessed it... repeat the process. Write out your gratitude reflections for the day. What happened in your day that filled you up, gave you hope, inspired a moment or moments of joy, pleasure, kindness. Again, start with just one and let it evolve from there.

Begin and end your day feeling grateful. On average, it takes more than two months before a new behavior becomes automatic (66 days to be exact). So, be patient with yourself. Practice, practice, practice. I do this each day and it has truly made all the difference.

When you are fully present in each living moment of your life, the here-and-now, it is easier to feel gratitude for the experience. This is, what I like to call Present Moment Practice (PMP). Have fun with it... be playful... celebrate gratitude.

ACCEPTANCE - GRATITUDE WHEN IT'S HARD

It can be challenging to feel any connection to gratitude when your life turns upside down, when you are suffering. Under these circumstances, feeling thankful for anything can feel so out of reach and, let's be honest, freaking impossible!

Gratitude comes from your capacity to be fully present in each living moment, what I call what-is-thinking. This requires healing yourself from what-if-thinking.

You may, at times, find yourself held hostage by your what-if habit...

- What if I don't recover?
- What if I fail?
- What if it hurts?
- What if I hurt somebody else?
- What if I am judged?
- What if I am let down?

- What if I am rejected?
- What if IT comes back?

All these prognostications of an undetermined future, of what may or may not be, undermine your efforts. And you have absolutely no control here. So, instead, what if you choose to live in the what-is moment. As in, right now, this second...

- I am enough.
- I am connected.
- I am grounded.
- I am curious.
- I am creative.
- I am optimistic.
- I am brave.
- I am resilient.
- I am growing.
- I am grateful.

In this way, we are making a conscious choice... we are taking control, despite the chaos that may exist within and around us... empowering equanimity... cultivating capacity through gratitude and acceptance.

ACTION

What are the behaviors associated with gratitude?

• Acts of Self-Love/Self-Care

- Accepting of ourselves, as we are, in this moment of our journey

- Honoring our bodies, as they are, in this moment, not how we think they should be or could be better, tomorrow or the next day

- Choosing to eat, hydrate, move, restore, and sleep healthily

- Playing and inviting joy

• Acts of Love

- Accepting of others, as they are in this moment of their journey

- Fostering aligned, nourishing relationships

- Setting healthy boundaries as an act of love, a form of respect for self and others

Exercise:

Take a little time, right now, to reflect upon and feel grateful for the peeps who have your back, no matter what. They are the ones by your side when you are at your very best and they remain by your side when you are at your very worst.

Now, grab your journal and write down the names of each person in your inner circle. Next to each name, write down why you feel grateful for their presence in your life. They continue to hold space for you, love, champion you with no judgment, while holding you accountable... not letting you get away with anything... keeping you honest... helping you own your shit. Cherish these humans fiercely, and when they find themselves in need of support, you know exactly where you will be... by their side.

• **Acts of Service:**

- To yourself

- To family and friends

- To community

- To mother earth

- To reconciliation

- To social equity and justice

When we are grounded in gratitude, when we are fully present, connected to our gifts... and YES, we all have them... only then are we able to truly show up and shine our light in the world, to make the difference we are meant to make.

Audio Recording: Access "Gratitude Meditation" in your RECLAIMED Library: https://bit.ly/accesslibrary

TO RECAP:

✓ You now know the 3 A's of Gratitude: Attitude, Acceptance, and Action.

✓ You recognize that gratitude is an attitude, a conscious choice.

✓ You are empowered with tools to enact gratitude, even when it's hard.

✓ You now have clarity around the behaviors associated with gratitude: Acts of Self-Love and Self-Care, Acts of Love in relationship, Acts of Service for the greater good.

✓ You now have another doorway, another opportunity to keep honing awareness, deepening connection, and taking mindful, purposeful action. Take a little time to reflect upon how a Daily Gratitude Practice may support the 3 Pillars of Pain-Free Living. Feel free to journal out your insights to fortify your knowledge and understanding.

✓ YOU ARE LEARNING TO MAKE A DAILY HABIT OF GRATITUDE.

When all else fails

Hang out in the sweet seat of gratitude

Joy happens here

Pleasure happens here

Love happens here

Enough happens here

Healing happens here

Living happens here

"You do not want to miss out on an opportunity to work with Julie! Guaranteed you will feel seen, heard, supported, and celebrated. At minimum, you will learn a new tool, invite a fresh perspective, or gain a helpful insight, as to how to empower your best health – in body and in mind. Julie weaves yoga, self-care, and hope into everything she speaks to, everything she does, and she shows you that anything is possible, including long-lasting healing and recovery."

- Reclaimed Mastery Client

CHAPTER 11

You're On Your Way!

Step Into Life

sometimes, we must...
step into discomfort
to find ease
step into dysfunction
to find function
step into chaos
to find peace
step into vulnerability
to find strength
step into sadness
to find joy
step into loss
to find connection
step into pain
to find healing
step into darkness
to find light

What a journey!

We have covered a lot of ground together.

My true hope is...

- You have learned strategies to empower your optimal state of being, in breath, body, mind, energy, and soul, in any given moment.

- You understand that robust whole health is the result of a daily, diligent practice in present moment awareness, connection, and action.

- You trust yourself to play safely in the realm of possibility.

- You are beginning to experience the freedom of living your life purposefully, with capacity, equanimity, and grace.

TRANSFORMATIONAL INSIGHT: Returning to a place of true joy may require several visits to the Lost and Found. Do not give up! Remain hopeful, be patient, trust, and persevere. Because one day, after its wayward journey, joy will be back, cheekily awaiting your arrival. It may turn up a little tired, tattered and bruised. It may feel different than you remember it, but it is unmistakably yours, freaking beautiful, and home at last.

KEY TAKEAWAYS:

1. Wellness is a function of our daily habits.

2. Aim to make the 3 Pillars of Pain-Free Living, Authentic Awareness, Compassionate Connection, and Aligned Action, the GPS System of your day.

3. All that you need to navigate this life exists within you. To access its power, see the previous point.

4. Whenever the body is misaligned, the nervous system recognizes it as stress.

5. To heal effectively and sustainably we must first feel safe.

6. Long-term healing is built upon on an intentional foundation, not a house of cards.

7. When all else fails, return to your breath.

8. Talk to yourself like you are the love of your life...YOU ARE.

9. Yoga should never hurt... EVER.

10. Asana (movement) is simply about making shapes that make sense and feel good in your body, in any given moment in time.

11. Meditation does not need to be hard or go on forever. Nor does it require you to empty your mind, levitate, or leave your body. It is one of the most effective ways to strengthen your first two pillars... Authentic Awareness and Compassionate Connection.

12. Fear, like all our emotions, serves a purpose. With discernment, we can learn to use fear to our advantage.

13. Gratitude springs from our capacity to be fully present in each living moment of our lives. It can be the game changer, particularly when the going gets tough.

Last thoughts…

'Feel-good' living is your birthright.

Be resolute in its pursuit.

You are worth it, and the world needs your magic.

Epilogue

Moving through healing and recovery is not a linear path. In fact, it can feel more like some sort of crazy-ass square dance that in no way resembles a square. One step forward, followed by two steps back, a dogleg left, and then spinning, lots of spinning!

In the beginning, there is no rhythm, no groove. It's just a free-for-all of overwhelming thoughts and feelings, not to mention exhaustion from the sheer effort of keeping it all flowin' and goin'. We can hang out here for quite some time, in some variation of this funky little Fox Trot, trying to make sense of it all. Some days we are rockin' it, and other days we are crashin' and burnin' in some sort of dramatic, not so graceful final act. When all is said and done, it looks and feels a whole lot like fetal position. Oh! Wait a minute. That's because it is! And it is right here, in this glorious heap of humanness, where we must catch ourselves... slow it all down... curl inward a little more, not to hide, but rather to hold ourselves even tighter, with deeper compassion, acceptance, and love.

There is no rush. We must do the inner work. We must give ourselves ample opportunity to reflect and remind ourselves that we are worth it. Perspective will come and life will feel good again. This is the practice. We reset and repeat as required.

With love,
Julie

> *We cannot become ourselves by ourselves.*
> *– Dr. Claire Zammitt*

Healing is not easy work,

but it is the best work
you will ever do.

A RECLAIMED CLIENT WITH THE LAST SAY...

"Grace. If you look it up in Webster's, the definition begins like this, " Unmerited divine assistance given to humans for their regeneration...". For me, meeting Julie Thayer was nothing short of an experience of serendipitous grace. I was introduced to Julie a bit less than a year ago through a friend. In hindsight, I view that meeting as a sort of holy encounter, the outcome of which was my decision to enter her Reclaimed Mastery program. 6 months later, I can tell you it's been one of the best decisions I've made in my life!

Back then, though you never would have guessed it by looking at me from the outside, I was in rough shape. I have had a lifelong struggle with depression and found myself, once again, winding my way through its dark inertia while simultaneously trying to manage something new - extreme bouts of anxiety and panic. They had come, seemingly, out of nowhere. I had been in months of physical therapy for back and hip issues, IBS was ruling my life, and I had just had a workup by a cardiologist after enduring a month of odd and deeply disturbing episodes of heart palpitations. The circumstances of my life could explain some of this struggle, but suffice it to say, my nervous system was screaming at me for help. I knew that if it had to scream at me much louder, I was potentially at risk of paying a much higher price. And I knew I needed help; I just had no idea what that help might look like. After oodles and gobs of doctors and therapists and adjunct modalities to no good end, I was about burned out. Then, enter Julie and her program. Serendipitous grace.

In these last few months since starting the program, I feel myself transforming, shifting, settling down, and becoming healthier in all layers of my being. The changes in me have progressed subtly but are increasingly noticeable to me and others around me. Julie speaks of being able to meet life and its challenges with more capacity and equanimity by developing and honing the skills we discuss, and that's exactly what's happening for me. The tools for doing so, on the surface, seem relatively simple - breath work, gratitude, self-awareness, values clarification, yoga... But I am here to tell you, there is profound in the simple. I have used the breath work to manage my way through some of the worst of my panic and anxiety, the gratitude practice to shift my perspective and focus (and it's true, what you focus on grows!), and the self-awareness to guide my steps day by day. The exercise of distilling that which I value down to three top values has been one of the most helpful things. I reflect daily on the values I identified, and they serve as an anchor when the seas of life get stormy. They have truly become a guiding light.

Once upon a time, I thought of yoga as bendy-pretzel moves with funny Sanskrit names that you did on a slim, rubbery mat. Yoga is that, yes, but I've learned it is also so much more! The self-awareness required and the concepts of "nudging edges" and "baby toe steps" (Julie's languaging) play just as well off the mat as they do on the mat. On the mat, Julie has been vitally helpful in supporting me with workarounds when my physical body just isn't up to the form of a pose. She's also taught me restorative poses to utilize for support in calming my overactive nervous system, and they have been immensely helpful! And all of this is only a portion of my experience! Bit by bit, week by week, thread by thread I am weaving together a tapestry of practices that I will be able to wrap around me for the rest of my days. Simple, daily, SUSTAINABLE, practices. Profound. I am so very grateful for the teaching in this program, for the courage and commitment I've been able to summon which has allowed me to accept, utilize and grow with it, and for Julie, who has reminded me of how truly wondrous life can be, and how utterly love can transform. I am different because of this work, and it has made all the difference... for me, for my relationships, for my life."

- Reclaimed Mastery Client

It has been an honor to walk with you.

- If this book has resonated with you and you wish to work with me further...
- If you are deeply committed to stepping into the driver's seat of your pain experience and reclaiming your life...
- If you know you will need ongoing support, accountability, and empowerment to ensure sustainable transformation...
- Then I invite you to book a free coaching call with me.

Take your breath back. Take your body back. Take your heart back. Take your mind back. Take your energy back. Take your soul back. Take your life back.

LET'S JOURNEY TOGETHER.

https://bookcallwithjulie.as.me/reclaimed

Bibliography

Claffey, Karen. Heaven on Earth Yoga Institute & IHYT Integrated Health & Yoga Therapy. Yoga Therapist Training Manual. 300 Hours Yoga Therapist Training. 500 Hours Yoga Alliance Registered. 2002 – 2013.

Cloud, Henry, and John Townsend. *Boundaries: When to Say Yes, How to Say No to Take Control of Your Life.* New York: Zondervan, 1992.

Government of Canada. "Mental-Health Anxiety Disorders." https://www.canada.ca/en/health-canada/services/healthy-living/your-health/diseases/mental-health-anxiety-disorders.html. Published July 2009

Johari, Harish. *Chakras: Energy Centers of Transformation.* Rochester, Vermont: Destiny Books, September 1, 2000.

Kaoverii Weber, Kristine. "Yoga Cosmology, Psychology & The Chakras." Workbook. Satva Health LLC, 2012.

Mikulic, Matej. "Value of U.S. nervous system disorders from 2014 to 2019." Statista. Health. Pharma & Medtech. Pharmaceutical Products & Market. https://www.statista.com/statistics/445671/us-nervous-system-disorders-market-size/. Published September 20, 2021.

Mood Disorders Society of Canada. "The Human Face of Mental Health and Mental Illness in Canada." Chapter 5, Anxiety Disorders. http://mdsc.ca/documents/Consumer%20and%20Family%20Support/Anxiety%20disorders_EN.pdf.

National Institute of Neurological Disorders and Stroke. "Brain Basics: Understanding Sleep." National Institutes of Health. https:// www.ninds.nih.gov/Disorders/Patient-Caregiver-Education/Understanding-Sleep. Published August 13, 2019.

Science Daily. "Waking just one-hour earlier cuts depression risk by double digits, study finds." https://www.sciencedaily.com/ releases/2021/05/210528114107.htm. Source: The University of Colorado Boulder. May 28, 2021.

Shah, Parita. "A Primer of the Chakra System." Chopra. https://chopra. com/articles/what-is-a-chakra.

The Mayo Clinic. Anxiety Disorders. Patient Care & Health Information. Diseases & Conditions. https://www.mayoclinic.org/ diseases-conditions/anxiety/symptoms-causes/syc-20350961.

About The Author

Julie Thayer: Yoga Coach - E-RYT 500, Women's Health & Trauma Specialist, Kind Movement Expert, Creator of RECLAIMED – The Mastery™, Contributing Author of a Bestselling Book, Mental Health Advocate & Self-Care Champion

Julie has been a fitness enthusiast all her life. An athlete in her early years, her motto was "Harder. Stronger. Faster!" and thus, her relationship with yoga was, shall we say, tenuous at best. A nagging curiosity compelled her repeatedly back to her mat, until she eventually began to embrace the idea less is more. And then she fell hard and fast for this yoga thing. Joyfully understanding that connection to breath, mindful movement, and kind alignment, supports the integration of the whole and inspires vitality in all the layers of ones' being. Julie is a firm believer in becoming the champion of your own self-care and she will inspire you to discover your own capacity to cultivate an optimal state of being through your personal yoga practice, both on and off your mat.

Having navigated her own healing journey from chronic physical pain, lifelong depression, and anxiety, Julie specializes in helping women successfully overcome their physical and/or mental-emotional pain and illness, to reclaim their lives, and return to empowered feel-good-living. Her passion for yoga, and a sincere desire to serve her clients, is the inspiration behind her signature program, RECLAIMED – The Mastery™. In this 8-month immersion program, Julie utilizes proven yoga and self-care strategies to propel sustainable whole health transformation for the women with whom she works worldwide. She is also a contributing author of the bestselling book, *Change MAKERS* – 20 transformational stories from women making an impact in the lives of others. In her chapter, Julie shares her story of overcoming deep depression and surviving suicide.

A little more about Julie: she completed her…

- RYT 200 teacher training at White Lotus Foundation in Santa Barbara, CA under the direction of Ganga White, Tracey Rich, and Sven Holcomb. It was a life-altering experience, to say the least.

- RYT 500 teacher training mentoring with Karen Claffey and the esteemed faculty of The Heaven on Earth Yoga Institute in Stoney Creek, Ontario. Julie's studies at Heaven on Earth focused upon Structural Alignment based upon Anusara Universal Principles of Alignment. This intensive training profoundly impacted Julie's deeper understanding of the power of yoga to both nurture and inspire one's mind, body, and soul.

  - Anatomy and Physiology, Yoga for Chronic Pain with Neil Pearson

  - Yoga for Cancer, End-of-Life and Chronic Illness with Jnani Chapman

- Yoga for Grief Relief, with Antonio Sausys

- Yoga Cosmology, Psychology and The Chakras with Kaoverii Weber

- LifeForce Yoga for Anxiety and Depression with Joy Bennett and Amy Weintraub

- Introduction to Ayurveda with Nitin Shah M.D.

- Yoga for Arthritis, Osteoporosis, and Fibromyalgia; Restorative Yoga and Yoga Nidra

• SUP Yoga Teacher Training/Paddle into Fitness Certification and Level 1 WPA SUP Instructor Certification with Gillian Gibree and Paddle Into Fitness

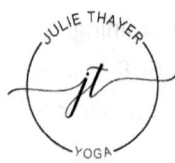
JULIE THAYER
jt
YOGA